K. A. Parker

July 6th, 1981

THE COLONIAL PHYSICIAN

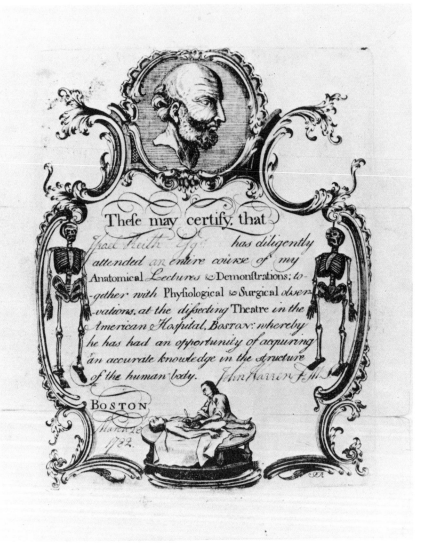

Anatomical lecture certificate engraved by Paul Revere

WHITFIELD J. BELL, JR.

THE COLONIAL

PHYSICIAN

&

OTHER ESSAYS

S H P

1975   SCIENCE HISTORY PUBLICATIONS   NEW YORK

First published in the United States by
SCIENCE HISTORY PUBLICATIONS
a division of
Neale Watson Academic Publications, Inc.
156 Fifth Avenue, New York 10010

© SCIENCE HISTORY PUBLICATIONS 1975
First Edition 1975
(CIP Data on final page)
Designed and manufactured in the U.S.A.

CONTENTS

ACKNOWLEDGEMENTS

We should like to express our sincere appreciation to a number of scholarly publications for granting us permission to reprint articles in this current volume. They are as follows: Bulletin of the History of Medicine, The Johns Hopkins University Press, "Portrait of the Colonial Physician," 44:497-517, 1970; Pennsylvania Magazine of History and Biography, "Philadelphia Medical Students in Europe, 1750-1800," 1-29, 1943; "John Redman, Medical Preceptor (1722-1808)," 81:157-69, 1957; William and Mary Quarterly, "Thomas Parke, Physician and Friend," 6:569-95, 1949; Johns Hopkins Press, "James Hutchinson (1752-1793)," 265-83, 1968; Annals of Medical History, "James Smith and Public Encouragement of Vaccination," 500-17, 1940; Bulletin of Cleveland Medical Library Association, "Benjamin Franklin and the Practice of Medicine," 9:51-62, 1962; Bulletin of the History of Medicine, "Lives in Medicine: Biographical Dictionaries of Thacher, Williams and Gross," 42:101-20, 1968; "Joseph M. Toner (1825-1896) as a Medical Historian," 47:1-24, 1973; University of Pennsylvania Library Chronicle, "John Morgan: Adventures of a Biographer," 53:213-23, 1951; Medical History Magazine, "Adam Cunningham's Atlantic Crossing, 1728," 50:195-202, 1955; Journal of the History of Medicine, "William Shippen's Introductory Lecture, 1762," 25:478-79, 1970; "Body Snatching in Philadelphia," 108-110, 1968; University of Pennsylvania Library Chronicle, "An Eighteenth Century American Medical Manuscript," 213-23, 1951; Journal of the History of Medicine, "Dr. James Rush on his Teachers," 19:419-21, 1964.

We should also like to express our appreciation to the New York Academy of Medicine for permission to reproduce the portraits of Redman, Shippen, Hutchinson, Gross, Thacher, Toner, and Morgan; to the American Philosophical Society for the portrait of Franklin; to the Frick Art Reference Library for the portrait of Parke, and to the Massachusetts Historical Society for the frontispiece. If the publishers have unwittingly infringed the copyright in any illustration reproduced, they will gladly pay an appropriate fee on being satisfied as to the owner's title.

INTRODUCTION

In 1939 Whitfield J. Bell, Jr. was a young instructor in American history at Dickinson College, his alma mater, and working for his Ph.D. at the University of Pennsylvania. For a paper on Latin-American history, he had been reading American newspapers from 1810 to 1820 and noticed an advertisement of the National Vaccine Institute signed by a Dr. James Smith. Such an institute on a national basis aroused his curiosity, as did the fact that Smith was a graduate of his own college, whose history was of particular interest to him.

That summer he had permission to work at the Welch Library and the Institute of the History of Medicine at the Johns Hopkins where he was given a warm and friendly welcome by Drs. Henry Sigerist and Owsei Temkin and by Genevieve Miller and Janet Koudelka, members of the staff. As Bell became familiar with the life and work of James Smith, he also became acquainted with the standard reference works in the history of medicine and, since he has always had a wandering eye when confronted by books, with some medical biographies and essays as well. Dr. Francis Packard, editor of the *Annals of Medical History*, published "James Smith and Public Encouragement of Vaccination" in 1940. This, the first paper of Whitfield Bell in the history of medicine, was not to be his last.

At this time he was writing his dissertation at Pennsylvania under Richard H. Shryock. Although Dr. Shryock had already published a number of papers and a book on *The Development of Modern Medicine: an Interpretation of the Social and Scientific Factors Involved* (1936), he was not directing his graduate students toward medical history and few of them had read his book. He was regarded more as a general social and cultural historian, and indeed Bell had chosen as his subject "The Social and Cultural History of Philadelphia during the American Revolution and Confederation." It was a natural choice. He was already aware that rich and extensive manuscript and archival material useful to his purpose was preserved in the institutions of Philadelphia—the Library Company, the American Philosophical Society, the Historical Society, the Society of Friends, and the Free Library. He had also made friends among the custodians of these collections as he would later among the private owners of diaries and letters he had a particular talent for locating.

As he moved deeper into his research, he discovered that many of the leaders in social reform in the city had been physicians and he perceived a close link between their scientific training and their humanitarian aspirations. He began to discuss aspects of medical history with Dr. Shryock, and it was at Shryock's suggestion that he wrote the paper on "Philadelphia Medical Students in Europe, 1750-1800" which appeared in 1943.

A few years later, in response to an editorial in the *Bulletin of the History of Medicine* urging the need for local studies in the field, Bell wrote "Suggestions for Research in the Local History of Medicine in the United States" (1945, *17*, 460-476). While he agreed with the editorial, he found much of the work that had been done in local history disappointing.

... When it has even failed to establish facts and fix chronologies the work has indeed been worthless. . . . To study a subject so narrowly is to leave it unenriched. No normal community but has its relations with other communities and their tides of opinion. History is more than chronology and more than annals. Specifically, in American medical history, too many researches have ignored the social and intellectual frame within which professional developments have proceeded. Because it is always concerned with persons, medicine cannot be regarded as significant apart from the other interests of men. The medical sciences and arts are not revealed and practised in a social vacuum. Their history cannot be written in an intellectual vacuum. (pp. 460-461)

In his own work Bell followed this good advice. Although he has shown obvious interest in the characters on the stage, he has never failed to provide both backdrop and motivation for the action. The title of his dissertation became "Science and Humanity in Philadelphia, 1775-1790." He then proceeded to prove a statement he had made in his "Suggestions"—"the whole medical history—and more—of a city or a generation can be illustrated and illumined by biographical studies of a group of doctors."

In 1954 he gave up his professorship to devote seven years to editorial work on The Papers of Benjamin Franklin at the American Philosophical Society and at Yale University. But since many of Franklin's friends—and regularly his collaborators in schemes for the public good—were physicians, these years contributed to Bell's knowledge of Philadelphia doctors and their part in social reform in the city.

He studied the early faculty of the medical school and eventually wrote a full-length biography of John Morgan (University of Pennsylvania Press, 1965) whose *Discourse upon the Institution of Medical Schools in America* laid down the principles of a sound medical education. He also wrote on William Shippen, Adam Kuhn, and Benjamin Rush and on important physicians in the Pennsylvania Hospital who were popular preceptors as well, such as John Redman and Thomas Parke. Like Franklin, Bell recognized it is not always the most brilliant minds in the world that carry on its work. In the fascinating re-creation of "Thomas Parke, M.B., Physician and Friend," he stated his thesis.

Neither great nor indispensable, he [Thomas Parke] was thus a man of the second rank. The world is filled with such people. Yet these men's lives have meaning. The Franklins and the Jeffersons on the one hand, the scoundrels and the killers on the other, are all well known; they crowd history's galleries. But it is the large body of unimaginative, undistinguished men of the middle sort who do most of the world's work. It is they who keep alive the ideas other men conceive and hold together the institutions other men create. They serve laboriously on committees, collect money for good causes, and preach and teach and write for the largest audience. They originate little; they transmit much. They are the ideal trustees, the perfect friends. They are the useful ones, like Thomas Parke. (pp. 569-570)

Each of these studies contributed something to the others until Bell had become so familiar with the life and people of eighteenth-century Philadelphia, particularly with those involved in medical and scientific activities, that he found himself considered something of an authority on its history.

At the annual dinner of the American Association for the History of Medicine in 1967 and in his Presidential Address to the Association in 1972 he paid tribute to the early biographers of physicians. Thanks to his consideration of James Thacher, Stephen Williams, Samuel Gross, and Joseph Toner as men, one can better appreciate their labors. Untrained as historians, busy in the practice of their profession, they nevertheless made a substantial contribution to medical history. Bell recognizes their limitations and their accomplishments. The biographies they provided, whatever their shortcomings, are often the only accounts available of many early physicians. Of the hundreds of users of these biographical dictionaries, Bell is probably one of the few to read them from cover to cover—an exercise which paid off in "a picture of medical practice and professional life not readily obtainable otherwise." He pointed out that these forgotten country physicians probably took care of a larger number of Americans than did the city physicians about whom more is known.

In his "Portrait of the Colonial Physician" (Fielding H. Garrison Lecture, 1969) Bell reminds us of other important considerations we are apt to overlook. "If it is misleading to describe the profession in colonial America in terms of only its most visible and articulate leaders, it is also deceptive to liken or contrast those leaders with the famous physicians in Europe. . . ." And he warned against comparing cities in America with principal cities in Europe.

> . . . There is no sound basis for comparing an American town of 30,000 inhabitants with the British capital with 500,000. The difference in size is a difference in kind. Philadelphia was not a lesser London, but a provincial center like Bristol, Manchester, Norwich, and Edinburgh, and bore somewhat the same relation to the capital that they did. The historian of medicine in the American colonial period, in short, should not only consider the careers of the nearly anonymous and almost forgotten physicians of the time, but also compare the profession in competence, organization, and reputation with the doctors of Essex, Norfolk, and West Country towns and villages.

The account of Whitfield Bell's first attempts to locate material for a biography of John Morgan reveals much of its author and his methods of research. It is one of the few things he has written in the first person. It tells something of his thoroughness and his way of ferreting out original material—it might be labelled luck, serendipity, or "the prepared mind." The seeming simplicity of his lively, vigorous prose is actually consummate skill in the use of the English language. But the clearest element of all is the enthusiasm he brings to research and everything he undertakes. The spur it provides to students, scholars, and friends who continually draw on his knowledge may well be of more help than his phenomenal recall of useful sources or the sound advice generously given. It is a tangible commodity in which the readers of this volume may share. We can be grateful to Neale Watson for gathering them together at a time when a friendly, humanistic interpretation of a number of citizens who lived within earshot of the Liberty Bell can only increase our understanding and admiration of our founding fathers.

Hamden, Connecticut   Elizabeth H. Thomson
30 January 1975

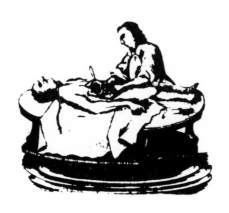

THE FIELDING H. GARRISON LECTURE *

A PORTRAIT OF THE COLONIAL PHYSICIAN

Unlike some of my predecessors in this series I cannot claim to have known Fielding H. Garrison; but I can—and do, most warmly—express my sense of grateful obligation to the Association for appointing me to this lectureship in his memory. In common with many others who have studied the history of medicine at any level, I cheerfully acknowledge my indebtedness to Colonel Garrison's published writings. Among the various subjects presented by Garrison lecturers in former years, there is probably none for which his *History of Medicine* or his essays do not contain useful information or helpful insights. About medicine in early America, to which, almost as an afterthought, he allotted a few pages at the end of his chapter on the Eighteenth Century, Garrison pronounced a chilling judgment: " There was no American medical literature to speak of until long after the American Revolution." [1] The dictum may well

* Delivered at the forty-second annual meeting of the American Association for the History of Medicine, Baltimore, Maryland, May 9, 1969.

[1] Fielding H. Garrison, *An Introduction to the History of Medicine* (Philadelphia: Saunders, 1914), p. 306.

daunt anyone who proposes to speak on that subject and time; but it should also have the salutary effect of keeping him from uttering superlatives and making unwarranted claims. In confession and avoidance I can only plead my topic is not American medical *literature*, but an aspect of the American medical profession: I shall sketch a few strokes in A Portrait of the Colonial Physician.

*   *   *

Biographies of only a small percentage of the physicians of colonial America have been written in modern times, critically, extensively, using all surviving data. Of an estimated 3,500 practitioners in 1775,[2] all but a few hundred are only names; of that small number fewer than 50 are usually cited in any description of the profession in the 18th century. Textbooks are content to mention Zabdiel Boylston and Benjamin Rush; general social and cultural historians add half a dozen more—Mark Catesby, John Mitchell, Lionel Chalmers, Joseph Warren; men who were often distinguished as much for careers in science or politics as in medicine. Practically all the names in any discussion of medicine in 18th century America are those of men who obtained European degrees, practiced in larger towns, founded medical institutions, or played prominent roles in public life, and, generally, can be cited as evidences of the maturation of American society and culture.

To sketch the profession in terms of its leaders and of institutions like Edinburgh University, the Pennsylvania Hospital, and the New Jersey Medical Society, however, is to draw a partial and distorted picture. The historian-biographer should take into account the hundreds of practitioners in towns and villages and in the countryside on scattered farms, not graduates of Edinburgh or founders of some medical society, who, for better or worse, formed the great bulk of the profession, provided the greatest amount of medical care, and gave the profession its prevailing tone. The names of Redman, Shippen, Rush, Physick, Coxe, and Wistar shine brightly in any catalogue of Philadelphia physicians at the close of the 18th century; but two-thirds of the 85 physicians and surgeons listed in the city directory of 1800 were not members of the College of Physicians or graduates of any medical school, and they are today mostly unknown. Who were George Alberti, David Bertron, Arthur Blaney, Bernard Frexo, Nathan Norgrave, Isaac Sermon, Albertus Shilack, John

[2] Joseph M. Toner, *Contributions to the Annals of Medical Progress and Medical Education in the United States before and during the War of Independence* (Washington, 1874), pp. 105-106.

Weaver, and, above all, Martha Brand of North Sixth Street, whose name appears not among the nurses, midwives, or surgeons, but as one of the physicians? [3]

If it is misleading to describe the profession in colonial America in terms of only its most visible and articulate leaders, it is also deceptive to liken or contrast those leaders with the famous physicians in Europe. It flattered Philadelphians and Charlestonians to think their cities at the close of the colonial period were smaller Londons; but I submit there is no sound basis for comparing an American town of 30,000 inhabitants with the British capital with 500,000. The difference in size is a difference in kind. Philadelphia was not a lesser London, but a provincial center like Bristol, Manchester, Norwich, and Edinburgh, and bore somewhat the same relation to the capital that they did. The historian of medicine in the American colonial period, in short, should not only consider the careers of the nearly anonymous and almost forgotten physicians of the time, but also compare the profession in competence, organization, and reputation with the doctors of Essex, Norfolk, and West Country towns and villages.

Addressing a local medical society at Sharon, Conn., which had named itself grandly " The First Medical Society in the Thirteen United States of America," James Potter in 1780 presented a highly colored picture of medicine in America in the preceding century and a half. He recalled to his audience all the familiar scenes and characters—the " howling and uncultivated wilderness," the "inhuman barbarians " who patrolled the woods " seeking to imbrue their hands in English blood," the " terrisonous accents of stern Bellona " drowning out " the agreeable voice of medical learning." In these circumstances the sick must resort to " some ignorant person who had only a superficial knowledge of the medicinal virtues of a few barbarous plants." When, in time, the harsh tasks of settlement and survival were completed and the colonists got more doctors and European drugs, they found they were no better off. A more terrible scene now opened—doctors, thoughtlessly following some manual or system, dosed and bled without reason or restraint, until the unhappy patient was " sent as it were dreaming out of the world." [4]

Though Dr. Potter's rhetoric owed something to patriotic emotion and

[3] *The New Trade Directory for Philadelphia, Anno 1800* (Philadelphia, 1799), pp. 130-132, 172.

[4] James Potter, *On the Rise and Progress of Physic in America: Pronounced before the First Medical Society in the Thirteen United States of America* (Hartford, 1781), pp. 4-7.

a need to measure the advances of his day by a past thought to be primitive
and debased, his views were by no means unique. Dr. John Morgan, at
the opening of the first medical college in the colonies in 1765, had said
similar things in hardly less impassioned prose. Uneducated physicians,
Morgan asserted, spread havoc " on every side," robbing husbands of their
wives, making wives helpless widows, increasing the number of orphans,
laying whole families desolate. "Remorseless foe to mankind! actuated by
more than savage cruelty! hold, hold thy exterminating hand." [5] And the
strictures of Dr. William Douglass of Boston still earlier in the century
are well known: "In general, the physical Practice in our Colonies,
is so perniciously bad, that excepting in Surgery, and some very acute
Cases, it is better to let Nature under a proper regimen take her Course
. . . than to trust to the Honesty and Sagacity of the Practitioner. . . .
Frequently there is *more Danger* from the Physician, than from the Distemper. . . ." The mode of practice, a native New England physician told
Douglass, was uniformly "bleeding, vomiting, blistering, purging, Ano-
dyne, &c. If the Illness continued, there was *repetendi* and finally
murderandi." [6]

Though many physicians were ill-trained, even untrained, there were
a good many of them; the colonies were not quite so destitute of doctors
as Potter described them.[7] In planned settlements a reasonably competent
medical practitioner usually accompanied each first shipload of emigrants.
At Jamestown Lawrence Bohune (d. 1621) was described by Captain
John Smith as "a worthy Valiant Gentleman, a long time brought up
amongst the most learned Surgeons and Physitions in Netherlands";
and he was succeeded by John Pott (d. *c.* 1642), "well practised in
Chirurgerie and Physique, and expert allso in distilling of waters " (an art
which helped undo him). Samuel Fuller (d. 1633) of Plymouth, "the
first regularly educated physician that visited New England," and a deacon
of the church, was called on to care for bodies and souls in Salem and
Charleston as well as in Plymouth. At New Amsterdam was George
Hack (fl. 1623-c.1665), a native of Cologne who was said to have
studied at the university of that city. Griffith Owen (1647-1717), who

---

[5] John Morgan, *A Discourse upon the Institution of Medical Schools in America*
(Philadelphia, 1765), p. 24.

[6] William Douglass, *A Summary, Historical and Political, . . . of the British Settlements in North-America* (Boston, 1749-53), vol. II, pp. 350-352.

[7] Biographical data in this lecture have been taken principally from the *Dictionary of
American Biography*, James Thacher, *American Medical Biography* (Boston, 1828),
and *Sibley's Harvard Graduates*. A facsimile edition of Thacher, with biographical introduction and bibliographical notes, was published by Da Capo Press, New York, 1967.

had practiced some time in Lancashire, came over with William Penn. These men, all among the first settlers, practiced medicine while they discharged a variety of civic functions and pursued private business interests, giving their neighbors as good medical care as was available in most of the villages of Britain and Germany. Perhaps the standard of medical care was relatively higher during the first period of settlement, when strong religious and political forces might act on a well-trained physician, than a generation or two later, when pressures and inducements to come to America were weaker.

By the second third of the 18th century the colonies were all, if hardly thickly settled, at least firmly established. " The first Drudgery of Settling new Colonies," Franklin had pointed out in 1743, was " now pretty well over." [8] The arts and sciences and the professions and trades that promoted them were emerging into steady growth; and the beginnings of specialization were at least noticeable. Such qualities of maturity also characterized the medical profession, which now displayed what Potter called " the first physical aurora in this American empire." [9] Far from being simple and accommodated to what some have supposed was the uncomplicated state of colonial society, medical practice was almost as complex and its practitioners nearly as varied as in the oldest nations of Europe.

First in prestige, though not in numbers or always in influence (since the opinions of the large number of mediocre physicians in a sense outweighed the judgments of a smaller number of well-trained doctors), were the " regular " physicians. The term cannot be defined precisely— it connotes a combination of formal preparation, ethical conduct, and demonstrated success in practice. Certainly graduates and students of a medical college—Leyden, Edinburgh, or Philadelphia, for example—were considered as having been " regularly " trained. There was never a doubt in Boston that James Lloyd (1728-1810) was a regular physician, for he had served a good apprenticeship and followed that with attendance on the lectures of Cheselden and Hunter in London; while in Philadelphia Thomas Parke (1749-1835), who had only a bachelor of medicine degree from the College of Philadelphia but had studied at Edinburgh, was always " Doctor " Parke, a member of the Hospital staff, and ultimately president of the College of Physicians of Philadelphia. American college graduates, like Robert Harris (1731?-1815), an alumnus of the College of New

[8] Leonard W. Labaree and others, eds., *The Papers of Benjamin Franklin* (New Haven: Yale Univ. Press, 1959-), vol. II, p. 378.

[9] Potter, *op. cit.* ftn. 4 above, p. 7.

Jersey, who served an apprenticeship of three or four years, might also be ranked among the regulars, for, like graduate M. D.'s, they had some theoretical base for practice. Finally, in the ranks of regular physicians were admitted some who, without formal professional or undergraduate education, had nonetheless served a good apprenticeship and practiced some time to general approbation. The case of the elder William Shippen (1712-1801) of Philadelphia is illustrative: he was an apothecary in the 1730s, but, as he acquired knowledge and experience, he gave up his shop and limited himself to the practice of medicine, with the result that in 1753, now reckoned one of " the faculty," he was elected a physician to the newly-founded Pennsylvania Hospital—the only one without a medical degree.[10] Needless to say, had Shippen still been the proprietor of the Sign of Paracelsus' Head, he would not have been chosen a Hospital physician.

On the whole the regular physicians were fairly well organized. They recognized one another, called one another into consultation, and in general strove to raise the standards of the profession, which they were agreed were shockingly low. In the 1740s Boston physicians met regularly in a " Physical Club." At Edinburgh in 1760 Virginia medical students, looking forward to practice, formed a club for mutual improvement in anatomy which obligated its members to work for the reform of medicine at home. All the members of the Philadelphia Medical Society of 1766 were regular physicians (though not all the regulars were members of the Society; but that is another story) ; and so were the New Jersey physicians who in the same year organized to raise the level of professional education and practice in that province.[11] Port and quarantine physicians were generally drawn from the ranks of regular physicians; and it was usually the regulars, like William Aspinwall (1743-1823) of Brookline, Mass., who organized inoculation hospitals and took the lead in most measures for the public health.

Had there been doctors who limited their practice to surgery or midwifery, they would probably not have been accepted as regular physicians. In fact, of course, there were few such practitioners. Medicine and surgery

[10] Whitfield J. Bell, Jr., "Medical practice in Colonial America," *Bull. Hist. Med.,* 1957, *31*: 445.

[11] Carl Bridenbaugh, ed., *Gentleman's Progress: The Itinerarium of Dr. Alexander Hamilton, 1744* (Chapel Hill: Univ. of N. Carolina Press, 1948), p. 116; Wyndham B. Blanton, *Medicine in Virginia in the Eighteenth Century* (Richmond: Garrett and Massie, 1931), p. 401; Stephen Wickes, *History of Medicine in New Jersey, and of its Medical Men* (Newark, 1879), pp. 43-49; Whitfield J. Bell, Jr., *John Morgan, Continental Doctor* (Philadelphia: Univ. of Pennsylvania Press, 1965), pp. 137-138.

were practiced by the same person, and he was acknowledged or rejected by the regular profession for reasons of education and conduct, not because of an arbitrary distinction. The distinction was, of course, jealously maintained in London; some British-born physicians sought to perpetuate it; and Dr. John Morgan wanted to establish it in America. But the proposal received little support. Even in Britain the separation of physicians and medicine from surgeons and surgery was not universally approved: Dr. John Gregory of Edinburgh denounced it as the source of much bad practice; and the book in which this sentiment was expressed was reprinted several times in the American colonies.[12]

For all that, some practitioners emphasized medicine or surgery without limiting themselves to it. A few, like Samuel Danforth (1740-1827) of Boston and James McClurg (1746-1823) of Williamsburg, simply had no taste for surgery—McClurg's biographer alludes to " the great delicacy of his nerves "—but others discovered they had a knack for the art, proved to be successful operators, and thereafter attracted more surgical cases than their brethren. They remained physicians nonetheless, unreservedly members of the regular profession. James Hutchinson (1752-1793) of Philadelphia was such a one. After graduating bachelor of medicine from the College of Philadelphia, on the advice of Dr. Fothergill who thought the city had enough physicians but needed a surgeon, Hutchinson studied anatomy and surgery in London; but on his return he practiced medicine as well as surgery and died prematurely, not of an infected surgical wound but of yellow fever caught from a patient. It was the same with midwifery. William Shippen, Jr. (1736-1808) of Philadelphia, James Lloyd (1728-1810) and his successor Isaac Rand (1743-1822) of Boston, and Hall Jackson (1739-1797) of Portsmouth, N. H., made obstetrics something of a specialty but were never considered anything but regularly bred physicians and ornaments of " the faculty."

Below the regular physicians was the vastly larger number of practitioners who had studied medicine for a winter or two with a more or less reputable country physician or, motivated in various ways, had taught themselves medicine and set up as doctors. Thomas Green (1699-1773) of Leicester, Mass., progenitor of a line of doctors, is said to have " received his first medical impressions and impulse " from a book given him by a British naval surgeon who was billeted at his father's and " took an interest in his [the lad's] vigorous and opening intellect." Young Green

[12] [John Gregory], *Observations on the Duties and Offices of a Physician; and on the Method of Prosecuting Enquiries in Philosophy* (London, 1770), pp. 40-46.

began practice in western Massachusetts with a gun, an axe, a sack, a cow, and a medical book; and, with the aid of that book and a knowledge of simples gained from the Indians, was soon able to treat the common maladies of his neighbors. However successful men like Green might prove to be, they seem to have had little professional esprit; indeed, living on the edges of the profession, sensitive to the limitations of their knowledge, they were a little inclined to scoff at the regular profession—though they usually saw to it that their sons who followed them into medicine got sounder training.[13]

For better or worse these men provided medical care of most kinds over vast areas. The best of them were conscientious, observant, devoted to their patients. They were not quacks; their common practice was hardly to be distinguished from that of the regularly trained; and in the end a few achieved more than local reputation. Dr. Alexander Hamilton of Annapolis, rarely disposed to think well of the medical practitioners he met on his gentleman's progress to and from Boston in 1744, was astonished to discover that Peter Bouchelle, "the famous yaw doctor" of Bohemia Manor, Md., was intelligent, knowledgeable, modest, and "not insensible of his depth in physicall literature." [14]

Often practicing in the same communities with such doctors as these, sometimes offering the only medical care available in remote settlements, were the clerical physicians. A clergyman was usually drawn into medicine out of local necessity. He might be the only educated person within miles, the only one with a handbook of domestic medicine, and therefore the only one able to diagnose and prescribe with confidence. There were always some in his flock who could not afford the charges of regular physicians or might fall into the hands of unscrupulous quacks; and again the clergyman, moved by Christian compassion, offered his help. "Since doctors are few and far between," explained the Lutheran patriarch Rev. Heinrich Melchior Muhlenberg (1711-1787), who cared for the bodies as well as the souls of the rural Pennsylvania Germans, "I necessarily had to take a hand myself." Called to comfort the sick and dying, the minister sometimes found that a drug would help as much as faith. "I asked my dear colleagues to unite in prayer to God for his life and true welfare,"

[13] Needless to say, the bleeders who worked on prescription and under direction of regular physicians, like Jacob Smith whom Dr. Adam Kuhn sent to the Drinker family during the yellow fever epidemic of 1798, were the menials of the profession, ranking near the bottom of the professional hierarchy, Henry D. Biddle, ed., *Extracts from the Journal of Elizabeth Drinker, from 1759 to 1807* (Philadelphia, 1889), p. 331.

[14] Hamilton, *Gentleman's Progress, op. cit.* ftn. 11 above, pp. 195-196.

Muhlenberg wrote of a visit to a sick man; "and in the meantime I prepared a few poultices. . . ." [15]

As practitioners of medicine, the clerical physicians should be considered along with other doctors. Some, with good training and wide experience, were in fact accepted as professional equals. The first president of the New Jersey Medical Society in 1766, for example, was Rev. Robert McKean (1732-1767), rector of St. Peter's Church, Perth Amboy, a missionary of the Anglican Society for the Propagation of the Gospel; while Rev. Jonathan Odell (1737-1818), of Burlington, N. J., was admitted to membership without examination, " being well known by many of the Society." Pastor Muhlenberg had acquired some medical knowledge during his student years at Halle; he regularly imported medicines from Germany and dispensed them freely among the sick poor of his extended parish. " Because . . . genuine *doctores medicinae* are rare in this country," he wrote, " I had to muddle through as best I could." [16] He respected the trained physicians in his neighborhood, generally calling them into any difficult case; and he had nothing but angry contempt for the empiricks, water-casters, and " quacksalvers " who gulled his people. He complained of the want of supervision of ministers and physicians alike. " We have only a very few properly educated and experienced doctors. Most of them are *empirici*, or at least *chirurgi*. The real *doctores* are not respected as they deserve to be, and are not used. The *empirici* are very busy and do a great deal of harm, for they are without supervision or order." [17] In the sickroom Muhlenberg performed with a resolute, no-nonsense attitude, even with a kind of grim humor, as when, summoned to offer spiritual counsel to a German physician or surgeon about to be hanged for receiving stolen goods, he called on the poor man to bear up and remember his anatomy—" death by strangulation was not much different from that by apoplexy." [18]

The combination of medical and spiritual advisor in one person held special risks. For one, the clerical physician found himself the recipient of all sorts of complaints and confidences—Muhlenberg once likened himself to a " privy to which all those with loose bowels come running from all directions to relieve themselves." [19] Another objection was that patient-parishioners were sometimes reluctant to pay the doctor's fees.

---

[15] Theodore G. Tappert and John W. Doberstein, trans., *The Journals of Henry Melchior Muhlenberg* (Philadelphia: Muhlenberg Press, 1942-58), vol. I, pp. 189-190.
[16] *Ibid.*, p. 168.
[17] *Ibid.*, pp. 381-382.
[18] *Ibid.*, vol. II, pp. 68-69.
[19] *Ibid.*, p. 268.

Christ, they pointed out, had healed the sick and sent no bills; why should not His ministers follow that holy example? [20]

It is not easy to distinguish empirics of little or no training from failed physicians from Europe, runaway surgeons of ships, quacks, and near-quacks. John Hall, who hobbled into Philadelphia on crutches in 1758, claimed to have studied under a famous lithotomist of Bristol, served some years in British vessels on the African coast and in the West Indies, and practiced a while at St. Kitts.[21] Who were William Henderson, " Practitioner in Physick and Surgery," Hendrick van Bebber, and Hugh Graham, who practiced in Philadelphia in 1732? What, one wonders, were the real qualifications of the Dr. Ludwig who came to Philadelphia in 1775 announcing that he had studied physic and surgery " at the most renowned Universities in Germany " and practiced " in the best Hospitals and Infirmaries " and in the army? [22] Some of these men were probably itinerants, who provided a good deal of the medical care available in the colonies. Many of this tribe " specialized " in particular diseases, as did James Graham (1745-1794), who offered his services " in all the Disorders of the Eye and its Appendages; and in every Species of Deafness, Hardness of Hearing, Noise, Ulcerations of the Ear, &c." [23] We may judge the quality of the care they dispensed by the same " Doctor " Graham, for he soon returned to London, where, opening a temple of health and Hymen, he offered the services of a " celestial bed " to barren and other couples.

" Quacks," wrote William Smith in his *History of the Province of New York* in 1757, " abound like Locusts in Egypt, and too many have recommended themselves to a full Practice and Profitable Subsistence." [24] With no medical societies, no licensing laws, and limited confidence that the regular profession could effect cures, the colonies were a hotbed of autodidacts. Dr. Hamilton encountered such a self-starter on Long Island: he had been a shoemaker until, "happening . . . to cure an old woman of a pestilent mortal disease," he began to be "applied to from all quarters," and gave up cobbling for physic—which he had " practiced " several years with sufficient success.[25] Another self-starting medic was

---

[20] Wickes, *op. cit.* ftn. 11 above, pp. 167-168.

[21] *Pennsylvania Archives*, 6th series, vol. XIV, pp. 285-287.

[22] *Pennsylvania Gazette*, March 15, 1775.

[23] *Ibid.*, June 30, Dec. 22, 1773.

[24] William Smith, *The History of the Province of New-York . . . to the Year M.DCC.XXXII* (London, 1757), p. 212.

[25] Hamilton, *Gentleman's Progress, op. cit.* ftn. 11 above, p. 91. On a trip from Annapolis to Boston in 1744 Dr. Hamilton encountered a sorry assortment of doctors—in Cecil

Philip George Sibble, the Anspach orderly to an officer billeted on Henry Drinker during the British occupation of Philadelphia in 1777-78: enticed by the prospect of a better life in America and the charms of the Drinkers' maid, he deserted, married the girl, and fled to Easton, Pa., where he set up among the Germans there as a physician and, in Mrs. Drinker's phrase, " sells medicine, and makes money fast, German like." [26]

Though they may not have made money fast, most regular practitioners in towns and larger villages appear to have had decent incomes; a few, by good economy and judicious investments, died rich. Country physicians usually lived on working farms—something Rush recommended for both personal and professional reasons: the produce would augment the physician's small cash income, while in his local character as farmer, he would more readily win the approval of prospective patients.[27] But country practice, Pastor Muhlenberg warned, was nothing for anyone unaccustomed to rural life—a townsman in such a situation would need some independent income to make ends meet.[28] On the other hand, ill-educated physicians, doctors in remote, poor and sparsely settled areas, quacks, and itinerants resorted to a variety of expedients to eke out a living. Young Benjamin Franklin's friend, John Browne (1667-1737) of Burlington, N. J., kept a tavern;[29] some marketed a panacea or other " cure "; a few stooped to crime. The poor remuneration of most physicians may have been a reason why so many eagerly accepted public offices and military commissions with their cash fees and regular salaries.

Economics was not the only reason, however. Prestige was another.

County, Maryland, a "greasy thumb'd fellow" who "professed physick and particularly surgery" and who extracted teeth "with a great clumsy pair of blacksmith's forceps"; at New York a drunken military surgeon of little education who damned Boerhaave for a fool and a blockhead; and at Albany physicians who chiefly prescribed local herbs and eked a living as barbers. One layman, fed up with doctors, told Hamilton that he had learned by experience to shun them as impostors and cheats and that "now no doctor for me but the great Doctor above." *Ibid.*, pp. 7, 53-54, 65-66, 179-180.

[26] Drinker, *Journal, op. cit.* ftn. 13 above, p. 279. I do not include as a category physicians found guilty of crimes, as Dr. Benjamin Budd of Morris County, N. J., was of counterfeiting in 1773. He received a pardon but was expelled from the New Jersey Medical Society. *New Jersey Archives*, 1st series, vol. XXVIII, p. 611, vol. XXIX, pp. 17-18, 28, 48, 62, 128, 335; New Jersey Medical Society, *Minutes and Proceedings* (Newark, 1875), p. 35.

[27] Benjamin Rush, "Observations on the Duties of a Physician, and the Method of Improving Medicine," *Medical Inquiries and Observations* (2nd edit., Philadelphia, 1805), vol. I, pp. 305-408.

[28] Muhlenberg, *Journals, op. cit.* ftn. 15 above, vol. III, p. 559.

[29] Fred B. Rogers, "Dr. John Browne: Friend of Franklin," *Bull. Hist. Med.*, 1956, *30*: 1-6.

The practice of medicine in colonial America did not rank with the law or the ministry in the intellectual endowments it required or, therefore, in the social rank it conferred. The parents of Charles Jarvis (1748-1807) of Boston would have preferred that he study law, but they thought him too shy and diffident, and so sent him into medicine, where, in fact, he had a distinguished career. Similarly, Samuel Holten (1738-1816) of Danvers, Mass., because of an early illness, could not attend college; but he could study medicine. The private knowledge of some doctors, that medicine had not been their first choice for a calling, understandably debased the profession in their own eyes. Not a few took up medicine after quitting the ministry, often for reasons of health, as did Joshua Brackett (1733-1802) of Portsmouth, N. H., and Aeneas Monson (1734-1826) of New Haven, Conn., who had been a chaplain in the French and Indian War. The explanation is that whereas the ministry required long hours of study and writing bent over a desk, the practicing physician might look forward to healthful days making his rounds on horseback. It is therefore not entirely surprising that a good many physicians left the profession, temporarily or permanently, as soon as better opportunity offered. Holten quit medicine completely after 16 years of practice; William Bradford (1729-1808) of Bristol, R. I., and Nathaniel Freeman (1741-1827) of Sandwich, Mass., both took up law; and a good many, during and after the Revolution, abandoned the profession for public service.

How did these physicians conduct themselves in their professions and as citizens? What did they do? What did the leaders and spokesmen of the profession say they did, or should do? Which qualities and achievements were particularly mentioned by contemporaries, both colleagues and patients, as worthy of praise or censure? What kind of man, in short, was the colonial doctor? Some answers to these questions may be found in contemporary biographical notices and eulogies and in admonitory lectures to medical students and addresses to physicians.

Here several warnings should be uttered. In the first place, the surviving data are neither representative nor impartial. One would like to have biographies, or significant materials for biographies, for all, or at least a substantial number of, practicing physicians of the period; but they do not exist. In general, we know anything about only the successful, locally prominent, or otherwise outstanding physicians. In the second place, many of the available data even about these outstanding figures provide no answers to the more penetrating questions we have about the profession, such as why a man went into medicine, or what his professional income came to. Finally, many judgments and opinions about the profession which we can find do not apply uniquely to colonial America. Complaints about punctuality of attendance, for example, are made at every time and place; they may be found in the Roman satirists and are not unknown in the 20th century. All that one can do is point to those qualities which seem to have been uppermost in the minds of those who commented on the physicians of 18th century America.

Medical students about to receive their diplomas were sure to be reminded, as young graduates always are, that they were only beginning, not concluding, their studies; that there was no substitute for the regular reading of medical literature, and that they must expect to spend laborious hours over books and journals if they would achieve success in practice and promote the dignity of the profession. Yet even as they addressed their hopeful juniors, the professors realized that few of the lads would ever own more than a shelf of books; that most of them would acquire skill in the profession, if at all, by experience and observation. Only here and there did a country practitioner manage to acquire a few professional works as they appeared. The fact that Joseph Orne (1749-1786) of Salem, Mass., read European journals was so unusual that biographers commented on it with approval and astonishment.

Foreign physicians in America were sometimes noticeable because they pursued a scholarly interest, often to the neglect of practice. Thomas Moffatt (d. 1787), a graduate of Edinburgh, and John Brett (fl. 1740), who had studied at Leyden and had a degree from Rheims, liked to peer through their microscopes, make little experiments, and discourse with strangers on the order, elegance, and uniformity of nature as displayed in the texture of animate and inanimate bodies.[30] More often than not, however, too notorious an interest in reading and experimental science excited popular suspicions that the doctor was a " notional " man, not quite sound or reliable in practice; at best, the interest was cited in disapproving tones as a sample of exotic eccentricity.

Far scarcer than books were opportunities for post-mortem examinations. Whenever you lose a patient, Samuel Bard counselled in 1769, " let it be your constant Aim to convert, particular Misfortunes into general Blessings, by carefully inspecting the Bodies of the Dead, inquiring into the Causes of their Diseases, and thence improving your own Knowl-

[30] R. W. Innes Smith, *English-Speaking Students of Medicine at the University of Leyden* (Edinburgh: Oliver and Boyd, 1932), p. 30; Hamilton, *Gentleman's Progress, op. cit.* ftn. 11 above, p. 156.

edge, and making further and useful Discoveries in the healing Art." [31] The advice was unexceptionable, but almost irrelevant, for opportunities almost never arose. Physicians in larger towns might occasionally examine the body of a criminal or suicide, but every project for more regular provision invariably evoked strong objections and even violent resistance. In the event, a physician who had ever examined a dead body at length, as John Bard (1716-1799) and Peter Middleton (d. 1781) did in New York in 1752,[32] was likely to cite the achievement to his credit thereafter and to gain reputation from it. But such post-mortems, though undeniably useful, were not so valuable as examining a deceased patient, as Bard had recommended.

Though reading medical texts and recording medical data were enjoined on the younger physicians and were usually mentioned approvingly by eulogists and biographers, too obvious a reliance upon texts in practice was something else. Far more praiseworthy was demonstrated capacity for accurate observations and sound thinking based on experience. Abner Hersey (1721-1787) of Hingham, Mass., " never wearied his mind with theoretical investigation, but contented himself with simple practical observations." Of Benjamin Shattuck (1742-1794) of Worcester County, Mass., his biographer wrote, " His knowledge was considerable, but his wisdom was superior to his knowledge. He knew much of the thought of other men, but was governed by a system formed from his own." Seth Bird (1733-1805) of Litchfield, Conn., was more distinguished for " acute sagacity, correct judgment, and talent at discrimination, than for learning or science "; his prescriptions were " simple, often inelegant, but always well adapted to the circumstances of his cases." William Douglass (c. 1691-1752), who had a Leyden degree, achieved an easy ascendancy over some young physicians of Boston by loudly rejecting formal systems and reminding his hearers that he had once called the great Boerhaave a mere compiler of books.[33] Empiricism, though a term of reproach among the learned, was, if successful, usually approved by the public, which liked its doctors to practice medicine with the same forthrightness they might bring to carpentry or farming.

Though medical care would probably have been better had physicians read and pondered more, it is also probably true that in some instances

[31] Samuel Bard, *A Discourse upon the Duties of a Physician* (New York, 1769), pp. 13-14.

[32] W. B. McDaniel, 2d, " The beginnings of American medical historiography," *Bull. Hist. Med.*, 1952, 26: 45-53.

[33] Hamilton, *Gentleman's Progress, op. cit.* ftn. 11 above, pp. 116-117, 131-132, 137-138.

their professional skepticism and rejection of professional nonsense—at its worst, their ignorance of notions—was a salutary check on uncritical acceptance of untested theories and extreme systems of practice. Marshall Spring (1742-1818) of Watertown, Mass., who " was no book man,"

appeared to learn more from the nature of the diseases of his patients by the eye than by the ear. He asked few questions. . . . He often effected cures by directing changes of habits, of diet and regimen. He used little medicine, always giving nature fair play. . . . He was . . . no friend to the profuse use of medicines, abhorred the tricks and mummery of the profession, used no learned terms, to make the vulgar either in or out of the profession stare.[34]

And Samuel Danforth (1740-1827) of Boston rejected bleeding when that procedure was everywhere strongly recommended: he believed it weakened the body's powers of resistance and had no effect on the disease.

Colonial American physicians do not appear to have treated the poor with much consideration or charity. At least medical students were so often adjured to treat rich and poor alike, deceased physicians were so often praised because they had done just that, that one must conclude that doctors gave scant thought to the plight of the sick poor. Ezekiel Hersey (1708-1772) of Hingham, Mass., was praised, as were some others, because he had never sued but one person, and that for £8 for two journeys of more than 60 miles each and a serious operation. It was long remembered to his credit that on a cold, snowy night he had responded to a call to a Negro woman eight miles away, saying to those who would have dissuaded him, " Whether black or white, she is of the human family and shall have my assistance." In Philadelphia someone whom Benjamin Rush described as " a trader in medicine " constantly refused to attend the poor and, if called on to visit them, would drive the messenger from his door with angry curses.[35]

This attitude should not be too surprising, for eighteenth-century men were great respecters of persons, and gentlemen had little knowledge of, and less sympathy for, the poor. Boerhaave, Fothergill, and Cullen, Rush would remind his students, were often seen coming out of the hovels of the poor—an edifying sight that vastly increased the esteem in which they were held by the wealthy.[36] But the argument apparently convinced few.

---

[34] Thacher, *American Medical Biography, op. cit.* ftn. 7 above, vol. II, pp. 98-99.

[35] Rush, " On the Vices and Virtues of Physicians," November 2, 1801, *Sixteen Introductory Lectures* (Philadelphia, 1811), pp. 125-126.

[36] Rush, " On the Means of Acquiring Business and the Causes which prevent the Acquisition, and Occasion the Loss of it, in the Profession of Medicine," November 4, 1807, *ibid.*, pp. 232-255.

To many physicians medicine was a trade, and, like other tradesmen, they preferred the custom of those who paid well and promptly.

Physicians were notoriously skeptics in religion; some were irreligious, a few even atheists. Educated in the sciences, trained to look for causes rather than to contemplate a First Cause, less certain than the clergy that God was always wise and merciful, having a clear notion of what their own intervention had achieved, physicians did not readily accept all the orthodox teachings of the church. At their worst, they had an offensive confidence in their own powers: to a patient who replied to the question how he was, " Much better, thank God! " a doctor retorted, " ' Thank God! ' Thank me; it is I who cured you." [37]

Skepticism was tolerated in the latter 18th century, but in the orthodox reaction following the French Revolution, physicians with rationalistic, deistical views were apt to be regarded as " singular," " wavering," " loose and unsettled." Too active skepticism might even injure a man's reputation. Nathaniel Peabody (1741-1823) of Plaistow, N. H., despite a distinguished career as a soldier, legislator, delegate to the Constitutional Congress, and speaker of the New Hampshire House, because he was a staunch republican and a " favorer of infidelity," died regarded by many of his virtuous neighbors as a " degraded character "—but in extenuation of this stern judgment it should be added that Peabody was also a great admirer and good judge of horse flesh and was once imprisoned for debt. Lemuel Hopkins (1750-1801) of Hartford, Conn., who admired Voltaire, Rousseau, d'Alembert, Volney, and other " infidel " writers, escaped condemnation because his character was otherwise irreproachable; he took up the Bible late in life and made a satisfying death. John Browne of Burlington, N. J., on the other hand, not only held, but propagated, unorthodox views—he parodied the Bible in doggerel verse—so that no matter what his professional competence might have been, he could hardly have expected to win much practice or personal reputation.

Many physicians were sensitive to the charge of irreligion, which they vigorously rejected in public, while in private accepting the criticism and offering in addresses to their fellow physicians and medical students elaborate reasons why a physician should be a believer. Rush, as usual, had a simple remedy: if physicians only attended church regularly, their religious faith would be sufficient. Even physicians who welcomed Sunday calls as an honorable excuse, could appreciate the economic and social benefits from regular church attendance. Rush went further still, taking

---

[37] Rush, " On the Vices and Virtues of Physicians," *ibid.*, p. 122.

the positive view that religious faith was an advantage in practice. It often supplied the want of professional skill, he advised; pious words from the physician were sometimes effectual where medicine failed. William Aspinwall (1743-1823) of Brookline, Mass., gave religious counsel at the sick-bed, as all clerical physicians did. "There is no substitute for this cordial in the materia medica," Rush declared firmly.[38]

A physician arriving at a patient's house after a long country ride in cold or wet weather was likely to be met at the door with a warming glass. John Green, Jr. (1763-1808) of Leicester, Mass., "was never known to yield to the well-intended proffer of that kind of momentary refreshment"; but others were. William McKissack (1754-1831) of Bound Brook, N. J., became a heavy drinker in consequence of this country custom;[39] while James Hurlbut (1717-1794) of Wethersfield, Conn., was addicted not only to ardent spirits but to opium as well.

He would not prescribe or even look at a patient in the last years of his life, till the full bottle was placed in his entire control, and daily replenished; it was his practice to take very frequently small potations, and at the same time swallow enormous quantities of opium. For many of his last years all the avails of his medical practice were expended in the purchase of this one drug; his spirits he obtained from his employers, which was a heavy tax, and he probably took as much opium as the most devoted Turk. He was rarely intoxicated, and when so much under the influence of alcohol as not to be able to stand, his mind would appear to be clear, and his judgment unimpaired.[40]

Though Dr. Hurlbut's excess was not typical of the profession, intemperance was. At least, older physicians constantly warned the younger against it. As late as 1826 David Hosack spoke out strongly on the subject, assuring his readers that the intemperate physician "under the influence of his daily inebriating potion" was "not a fancied picture." On one surviving copy of Hosack's address a proper Philadelphian penned a refutation. "I have never known a drunken physician in Penn-

---

[38] *Ibid.* See also John P. Batchelder, *On the Causes Which Degrade the Practice of Physick* (Bellows Falls, Vt., 1818), p. 4. The "undevout" physician in Batchelder's view simply was "mad," and if he was guilty of infidelity, it was because he indulged in some vice incompatible with religion.

[39] Andrew D. Mellick, Jr., *Lesser Crossroads*, Hubert G. Schmidt, ed. (New Brunswick: Rutgers Univ. Press, 1948), pp. 343-344.

[40] Thacher, *American Medical Biography, op. cit.* ftn. 11 above, vol. I, p. 309. Thomas P. Jones, *Charge to the Graduates in Medicine at the . . . Columbian College, D.C.* (Washington, 1830), p. 7, urged physicians to cultivate intellectual traits; one result would be that they would not succumb to "the temptations to which the Physician, and particularly the country practitioner, is exposed . . . that of drinking stimulating liquids" —the greatest and most baneful of his temptations.

sylvania," wrote Peter S. DuPonceau and then added significantly: "The possibility of the existence of a *drunken* Physician, should never have been admitted. It will injure this Country abroad and make foreigners believe that drunkenness is a common vice among our Medical Men." [41]

Except in times of epidemic, most physicians, especially those in small towns and the country, were probably not very busy; and their attendance on patients was marked by the same casual and leisurely pace that characterized rural life generally. Promptness and punctuality were unusual; at least they were constantly enjoined on young graduates by their professors and mentioned to the credit of every physician who observed them. Equally appreciated, wherever present, was a quiet manner, kindliness, and sensitive feeling for the patient and his family. Not a few practitioners, since they had not had the advantage of genteel rearing or of a college education, seem to have been rough, coarse, and abrupt; some even cultivated such a manner. Rush cited one physician who, being called to attend a very sick man, was urged to hurry because the patient was dying. "Then I can do him no service," the doctor replied. "Let him die, and be damned." [42] Vulgar, offensive, unmannerly were adjectives often applied to practitioners by those who had been better bred; we can only guess what their patients must have thought of them.

Professions have their badges and regalia; and physicians were no different from others. London practitioners affected large wigs and goldheaded canes, often bore themselves in a ridiculously stately manner, and spoke with absurd solemnity. Though there was less of this sort of thing in America, the tendencies were there, and Rush and others warned their students against them. Singularity in dress, manners, and speech, Rush declared, was "incompatible with the simplicity of science, and the real dignity of physic. There is more than one way of playing the quack." [43] There was indeed. Benjamin Waterhouse carried a gold-headed cane, but that was at the end of his life. A physician whom Dr. Hamilton met at Wrentham, Mass., dressed outlandishly in a weatherbeaten black wig, an old striped collimancoe banian, an antique brass spur on his right ankle, and a pair of thick-soled shoes tied with points [44]—but this was probably New England eccentricity rather than a claim to professional

[41] David Hosack, *Observations on the Medical Character* (New York, 1826), pp. 23-24. DuPonceau's commentary is in the American Philosophical Society copy.

[42] Rush, *Sixteen Introductory Lectures, op. cit.* ftn. 35 above, p. 125.

[43] Rush, *op. cit.*, ftn. 27 above, vol. I, p. 391.

[44] Hamilton, *Gentleman's Progress, op. cit.* ftn. 11 above, p. 148. A calamanco banian was a loose woolen gown. The gown (or shirt or jacket) was of Indian origin; but calamanco is a fabric of European manufacture.

notice; as was the behavior of Samuel Savage (1748-1831) of Barnstable on Cape Cod, who on the approach of the stage used to clamber atop a large boulder at the entrance to the village and cry out that he was a physician and surgeon.

The most important event in the life of every physician alive in 1755 was the American Revolution. Colonel Garrison declared that it was " the making of medicine in this country." [45] Like the French and Indian War before it, the Revolution afforded apprentices and young doctors an exceptional school of experience; it brought them into association with better trained men, inspired some to undertake further study—surgeon's mates were released from duty during the winter to attend medical lectures at Philadelphia—and provided observant physicians with materials for the medical communications that would at last make American medical literature, in Garrison's phrase, worth speaking about. The war and the efforts thereafter to establish and maintain effective governments also offered opportunities for profit, promotion, and new careers. It was perhaps to be expected that the great majority of physicians should support independence sooner or later. Those who did not, unless they made themselves singularly obnoxious, were generally unmolested or, if proscribed, were allowed, like John Jeffries (1744-1819) of Boston and Adam Kuhn (1741-1817) of Philadelphia, to return afterwards and resume practice. But it is a little surprising to mark how many neglected or abandoned their practices to answer to civil or military calls. In that republican era, of course, service to the state was the most urgent obligation of all; but the excitements of war and politics probably seemed more alluring in human terms than the humdrum of medical practice.

The doctors responded even before the first shots. Samuel Prescott (1751-1777) of Concord, Mass., son and grandson of physicians, completed Paul Revere's ride. Next morning several doctors appeared on the battlefield between Concord and Boston, not as surgeons, but as minutemen carrying rifles. Many wished to continue to serve in the field, though most were persuaded to accept appointments in the military hospitals by none other than Joseph Warren (1741-1775) of Boston, who did not take his own advice and was killed with the fighting troops at Bunker Hill. Other physicians, like Edward Hand (1744-1802) of Lancaster, Pa., William Irvine (1741-1804) of Carlisle, Pa., John Brooks (1752-1825) of Reading, Mass., Hugh Mercer (c. 1725-1777) of Fredericksburg, Va., and John Beatty (1749-1826) of Princeton, N. J., received

[45] Garrison, *History of Medicine, op. cit.* ftn. 1 above, p. 307.

commissions in the army and led troops in battle with success and distinction. Others, like the elder Josiah Bartlett (1729-1795) of Kingston,
N. H., who had been colonel of a regiment in the French and Indian
War, served principally in civil offices: he was in succession a member
of the provincial legislature, a justice of the peace, a delegate to the
Continental Congress, chief justice of New Hampshire, United States
senator, and governor of New Hampshire. Nathaniel Freeman of Sandwich on Cape Cod seems to have laid aside all practice for the duration
of the war. Jonathan Elmer (1745-1817) of Bridgeton, N. J., known in
medical-historical annals as a member of the first medical graduating class
at the College of Philadelphia, preferred politics to practice and from 1772
onwards was almost constantly in public office. So was Thomas Henderson (1743-1824) of Freehold, N. J., who began as a member of the Mon-
mouth County Committee of Observation on the eve of the Revolution,
served in the war as an officer and thereafter in the state assembly, on
the bench, and finally as a member of Congress.

The Revolution, Benjamin Rush wrote soon after the close of the war,
" rescued physic from its former slavish rank in society." Certainly many
doctors had demonstrated what they could do as patriotic men of affairs.
Some were revealed as the natural leaders of the community, freer than
the clergy to accept most kinds of public service. The popular esteem
thus gained for the profession Rush was determined to preserve. He
used to exhort his students thereafter to have " a regard to all the interests
of your country," informing the nation about useful arts and seizing
opportunities to diffuse useful knowledge and sound opinions of every
kind. Doctors no less than others should speak out on public questions [46]
Rush himself exemplified his lesson. In time, however, as the profession
became better organized and more respected for professional achievements,
and as more persons of other professions came forward, the physicians
dropped out of public life. Rush himself in his latter years confided to
Hosack that he thought he had spent too much time in concerns outside
his profession. And Hosack declared that the legislatures of the nation
would be better off if physicians were barred from election to them.[47]

It would be reasonable to expect that the infusion of physicians into the
legislatures and the courts of the new states would have benefited the
profession. Ought not these doctors-turned-legislators have taken an informed interest in measures for the public health? Might they not have
been expected to take a lead in, or at least give support to, enacting

[46] Rush, op. cit. ftn. 27 above, p. 393.
[47] Hosack, op. cit. ftn. 41 above, pp. 6, 18.

licensing laws and establishing standards of admission to practice? Ought it not have mattered in the councils of the state that they were or had been physicians? It does not appear to have done so. The explanation may simply be that most of the doctors in public service were not outstanding physicians (they were physicians who were otherwise outstanding); many had withdrawn from medicine into politics early in life; and, by the time they had power to do something for the profession, they hardly thought of themselves as physicians at all. The title " Doctor " signified a profession and for some a modest social position; it did not mean influence in the state medical society; and most of the medical statesmen preferred to be addressed, as soon as they earned the right, as " General," " Judge," or " Governor."

Despite its palpable effects and influence on American life and thought, the American Revolution hardly marks a clear breaking point in the conditions of medical practice and of the profession in America. Many physicians who had read medicine and begun practice before 1775 did not retire until the 1820s. Able and ambitious young men continued to go to London and Edinburgh and did so in greater numbers than before the war. Ill-educated physicians were as common after 1790 as before; ministers accepted responsibility for the sick; quacks flourished everywhere —and sometimes organized schools and issued diplomas. The same advice and warnings that Samuel Bard and Benjamin Rush gave their students were being given 40 years later by Hosack, John Godman, and others.[48]

Yet if the war itself had made little difference, time had. There had been no medical school in the British American colonies before 1765; at the end of the century there were several, and it was not unreasonable that the citizens of a long-established village should expect to be treated by a doctor with formal medical training. Medical journals were appearing and, thanks to improving postal service, physicians in even remote places could receive them. Medical literature in the 18th century may have been, as Colonel Garrison asserted, hardly worth talking about; but in the early years of the 19th century there would be the work and writings of Elisha Bartlett, William Beaumont, Daniel Drake, William E. Horner, Philip Syng Physick, Wright Post, Samuel G. Morton, Nathan Smith, John Warren, and Caspar Wistar—as well, of course, as of hundreds, thousands, of undistinguished, forgotten, but typical practitioners, the counterparts in 1820 of the Aspinwalls, Birds, Greens, Herseys, Ornes, Springs, and even Martha Brands of an earlier generation.

[48] See, for example, John Godman, *Professional Reputation. An Oration delivered before the Philadelphia Medical Society* (Philadelphia, 1826), as well as the essays of Hosack and Batchelder cited above.

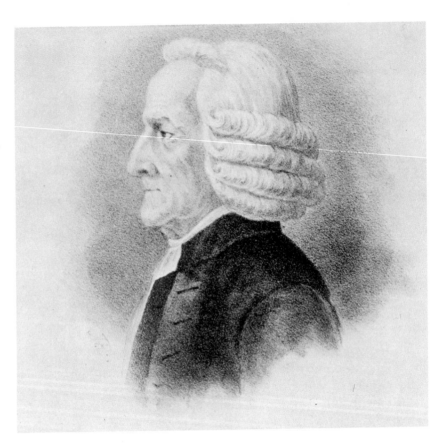

JOHN REDMAN

John Redman, Medical Preceptor
1722-1808

IN HIS dark broad-skirted coat, his German jack boots, and a hat that flapped before and was cocked up smartly behind, mounted on a fat little swish-tailed horse, Dr. John Redman, president of the College of Physicians of Philadelphia, must have struck some of his fellow citizens in 1800 as a curious survival from an earlier, simpler age.[1] To most of his professional colleagues, many of whom could not remember the time when Redman was fully engaged in active practice, he was a venerable relic who had known some of the first settlers of Philadelphia and had practiced medicine in the city before there was a hospital or anyone even dreamed of a medical school. At the opening of the nineteenth century he was in fact a very old man who had viewed the practice of medicine in Philadelphia through sixty years, seen medicine and the medical profession change, and helped make some of the changes. Odd though he may have seemed in his old flapping coat and full-bottomed wig, no one who knew John Redman laughed when he cantered by. To them— his patients, colleagues, coreligionists of the Presbyterian church— he was the *doyen* of the medical profession in Philadelphia.

Born in Philadelphia on February 27, 1722, educated at William Tennent's Log College on the Neshaminy, young Redman was apprenticed to able but ill-humored Dr. John Kearsley, Sr.[2] He was thus a member of that generation which saw far-reaching changes in

---

1 John F. Watson, *Annals of Philadelphia, and Pennsylvania, in the Olden Time* . . . (Philadelphia, 1881) II, 382. Everyone interested in Redman must be indebted to the researches of Dr. William N. Bradley of Philadelphia; his notes, including copies of many of Redman's letters, carefully organized and neatly mounted in two great volumes, are in the College of Physicians of Philadelphia, and are hereafter cited as Bradley. A painting and a silhouette of Redman are also in the College.

2 [Benjamin Rush], "Memoirs of the Life and Character of John Redman, M.D.," *Philadelphia Medical Museum*, V (1808), [49]-[56], is the principal source of biographical data, but must be used with caution, especially on Redman's views of practice. See also William S. Middleton, "John Redman," *Annals of Medical History*, VIII (1926), 213-223.

the education of doctors and the status of physicians. When the second third of the eighteenth century opened, all but a handful of physicians in America were either native Americans trained as apprentices to older doctors, or else self-taught; or they were men recently come from Europe, most of them of dubious qualifications, many of them adventurers and quacks, who stayed a year or two and then moved on. Among such Philadelphia practitioners in 1748, for example, the year in which John Redman received his degree at Leyden, were persons named John Andrews Zwiffler, John Rowen, Spitzer, Anthony Noel, and Matthias Brackel Vanderklüyt. Native-born Americans had not yet begun to go abroad for medical training, and nowhere in the colonies was formal instruction offered.

Thirty years later much of this had changed. Then the leaders of the profession in America, especially in the middle and southern colonies, were men with degrees from Edinburgh, Leyden, or Rheims. Physicians with such training strengthened and improved the quality of the apprenticeship system, which remained the common pattern of medical instruction. In several colonies and cities medical societies were formed to guard and raise the standards of the profession and to exchange medical knowledge. A few individuals, like the elder William Shippen, experienced the changes in a personal way: as a drug seller in 1730 he advertised himself simply "William Shippen, Chemist"; within twenty years he had joined Kearsley, Thomas Graeme, Phineas Bond, and six others in signing a public statement by the "practitioners of physic" of the city.[3] And in 1765 John Morgan and William Shippen, Jr., products of the apprenticeship system, but also graduates of Edinburgh, established at the College of Philadelphia the first regular medical school in British North America.

Having completed a rigorous apprenticeship with Kearsley, probably in 1743 or 1744 (he was still an apprentice on July 3, 1742, when he purchased a copy of Horace from Benjamin Franklin[4]), provided with a letter of recommendation from his master, Redman left Philadelphia and commenced to practice in Bermuda. After a short time, however, with an inheritance from his father and a loan from

3 *Pennsylvania Gazette*, May 18, 1749. The others were Christopher Witt, Lloyd Zachary, Samuel Preston Moore, Peter Sonmans, Richard Farmar, and John Kearsley, Jr.
4 Benjamin Franklin Ledger D (1739–1748), 157, American Philosophical Society.

Chief Justice Allen, perhaps on advice from Phineas Bond, who had been a student there in 1742, he enrolled at Edinburgh University in October, 1746. The great age of the Edinburgh medical school was just opening, and Redman was in the first generation of Americans to study there. He attended the lectures of Alexander Monro *primus* on anatomy and physiology and those of Charles Alston on materia medica, and probably also attended clinical lectures at the Royal Infirmary, which John Rutherford inaugurated that year.[5]

The second winter, 1747–1748, Redman spent at Leyden, whose university still glowed from the luster Boerhaave had given it. Here Redman studied anatomy, surgery, and midwifery under Boerhaave's student and collaborator, Bernhard Siegfried Albinus, and medicine with Jerome David Gaubius, Boerhaave's successor in the chair. As his dissertation Redman presented a subject in obstetrics— miscarriage. He dedicated it to Kearsley and Judge Allen and closed it with a prayer: "God grant that my studies and labors may be directed to the glory of his name, and to the welfare of my neighbors." Albinus was his sponsor in the final examination, and Redman received his diploma as a doctor of medicine on July 15, 1748.[6]

Both at Edinburgh and Leyden, however, Redman's work was bookish and largely theoretical. For practical experience and observation Redman is said to have visited the Paris hospitals after leaving Leyden, and in the winter of 1748–1749 he walked the wards at Guy's in London. From the attending physicians of that ancient foundation he received a testimony to his "great application."[7] In London a friend gave him a copy of Sydenham's works; on the flyleaf the donor inscribed the lines from Pope's *Temple of Fame* which end:

[5] His notes of Alston's materia medica are in the College of Physicians, and of Monro's anatomy and physiology, in the National Library of Medicine (formerly Armed Forces Medical Library), Cleveland. A list of students and apprentices made by Monro gives the name of J. Redman and his payment of a fee of three guineas on Oct. 29, 1746. L. W. Sharp to W. N. Bradley, Aug. 10, 1948, Bradley, I, 53-A.

[6] Redman, *Dissertatio medica inauguralis de Abortu* (Leyden, [1748]). The Album Studiosorum at Leyden shows that Redman enrolled as a student on Oct. 6, 1747. Curators of the University to W. N. Bradley, Aug. 17, 1948, Bradley, I, 53-C. See also R. W. Innes Smith, *English-Speaking Students of Medicine at the University of Leyden* (Edinburgh, 1932), 191. Redman's diploma is in the College of Physicians.

[7] [Rush], "Memoirs," *Philadelphia Medical Museum*, V (1808), [49]–[50]. The certificate is dated Feb. 21, 1748/9.

Unblemish'd let me live or die unknown;
O, grant an honest fame, or grant me none![8]

In the spring or summer of 1749 Redman returned to Philadelphia;
in November he purchased a Pennsylvania fireplace from Franklin[9];
and, thus re-established in his native place at the age of 27, he left it
seldom, and never for long periods, during the remaining sixty years
of his life.

Within three years Redman had acquired such a reputation in
Philadelphia that, with Thomas Graeme, Thomas Cadwalader, and
Charles Moore, he was asked to serve as a consulting physician in the
newly established Pennsylvania Hospital.[10] In 1756 he was com-
missioned a surgeon in Captain Vanderspiegel's Independent Company of Volunteers, although he served but briefly and probably
never left the city.[11] When Benjamin Rush came as an apprentice to
his house and shop in 1761, John Redman was said to have enjoyed
for ten years one of the largest medical practices in the city.[12] Though
for his health's sake he eventually gave up obstetrics and, some time
after 1765, surgery as well,[13] his income was substantial. He managed
it well, lived in great comfort, with a house in North Second Street
and a country place a few miles from town,[14] and retired after thirty
years' practice. He kept his shop, however—Washington bought
some articles there before returning to Mount Vernon in 1797—and

8 The volume is *Opera Medica* (Geneva, 1716); it was presented to the College of Physicians
by Redman. The inscription is dated Feb. 16, 1748/9. Almost forty years later Redman spoke
of himself in similar terms in his inaugural address as president of the College. He had never
had, he asserted, "great desires of exaltation above the middle state, nor higher ambition than
to conduct therein rather with integrity and usefulness than eclat." W. S. W. Ruschenberger,
An Account of the . . . *College of Physicians of Philadelphia* . . . (Philadelphia, 1887), 180.

9 Franklin Ledger D (1739–1748), 157.

10 Thomas G. Morton and Frank Woodbury, *History of the Pennsylvania Hospital* (Philadelphia, 1895), 28.

11 Robert Hunter Morris, Commission, Apr. 6, 1756, photostat, Bradley, I, 54, 55.

12 Benjamin Rush, *Autobiography*, ed. by George W. Corner (Princeton, N. J., 1948), 38.

13 In the certificate he gave his apprentice Samuel Treat on Sept. 1, 1765, Redman declared
that for nearly four years the young man had been "constantly employed in the practice of
Physic and Surgery under my care. . . ." Stephen Wickes, *History of Medicine in New Jersey*
. . . (Newark, N.J., 1879), 102.

14 Redman to Rush, Apr. 4, 1767, speaks of the building of his country house. Rush Manuscripts, XXII, 10, Library Company of Philadelphia. George Washington drank tea there on
July 9, 1787. *Diaries*, III, 227. See also Redman to Elizabeth Graeme Ferguson, June 5, 1776,
and Redman to John Nicholson, Oct. 15, 1799, The Historical Society of Pennsylvania
(HSP); and Redman to unnamed correspondent, July 25, 1772, typed copy of manuscript in
possession of Capt. F. L. Pleadwell, Honolulu, Bradley, II, 209. Redman's estate was valued in
1811 at $43,042.48. "Account of the Executors of the Will of John Redman, 1811," HSP.

when he was past eighty he was trying a new Indian herb and joined his colleagues in a public recommendation of vaccination as "a certain preventive of the small pox."[15]

Such a rush of business made it necessary for Redman to accept apprentices. Aspiring students, on their part, looked to Redman's shop as one of the best places in the city to receive good instruction and varied medical experience. He never took more than two apprentices at a time, and sometimes had but one—a limitation which, though it made Redman work more, doubtless made his students work harder too, and so promoted their education. Rush, who was recommended to Redman by President Davies of Princeton, remembered that in the five and a half years of his apprenticeship he was absent from his master's business only eleven days "and never spent more than three evenings out of his house." Rush kept Redman's books, and when the older man was ill or out of town, the whole burden of his practice fell on him.[16]

Redman gave his pupils Boerhaave and Sydenham to study, had them abridge Van Swieten's Commentaries, encouraged them to keep a commonplace book to record observations from his practice. He let young Benjamin Duffield copy his notes of Monro's lectures; his grandson John Redman Coxe filled a notebook with copies of his miscellaneous letters and papers on yellow fever.[17] Rush gratefully and warmly spoke of his master as unrivaled "in everything that's good." "I have experienced kindness from Dr. Redman I had little reason to expect," he continued. "I have ever found in him not only the indulgent master but the sincere friend and tender father."[18]

15 Rush to John Redman Coxe, Jan. 16, 1796, L. H. Butterfield, ed., *Letters of Benjamin Rush* (Princeton, 1951), II, 769; Redman to Rush, Sept. 25, [1804], Rush Manuscripts, XXII, 9; Cecil K. Drinker, *Not So Long Ago* (New York, 1937), 101–102; "Washington's Household Account Book, 1793–1797," *The Pennsylvania Magazine of History and Biography (PMHB)*, XXXI (1907), 346.

16 Rush, *Autobiography*, 37–38.

17 The notebooks of both Duffield and Coxe are in the library of the College of Physicians.

18 Rush to Ebenezer Hazard, May 21, 1765, Butterfield, I, 13. A few years later, however, when Rush wanted Redman's support in his application for the post of professor of chemistry in the College of Philadelphia and Redman thought he should wait until he returned home, advising him to bring with him a certificate of his qualifications "as it will be more honorable to you, and the Colledge, to ground their Election thereon," Rush spoke angrily of his preceptor. Rush to John Morgan, Jan. 20 and July 27, 1768, Butterfield, I, 49–50, 62; Redman to Rush, May 12, 1768, Rush Manuscripts, XXII, 11; Redman to Rush, n.d., *ibid.*, 19. The ill feeling on Rush's part—there was never any on Redman's—soon evaporated, and Rush subsequently dedicated the first volume of his *Medical Inquiries* to Redman, and Redman put his grandson in Rush's shop to study medicine.

Benjamin Waterhouse, writing in 1790, when he was a professor in the Harvard Medical School, assured him that his kindness sixteen years before was "still fresh in my memory."[19]

Redman reciprocated the tenderness of his apprentices and young friends. He rejoiced in their success, advised and encouraged them like a wise father, called them with affectionate pride his "professional children." "As it is no small gratification to my ambition, to have been instrumental in initiating you and other young gentlemen of reputation into that part of life which is most important," he assured one, "so it is & will be one of the greatest joys of my increasing years, & declining age, to see you prosper. . . ."[20] Each year he sent Rush—his "justly respected, & much esteemed Christian friend & medical son"—a friendly Christmas or New Year's greeting.[21]

Boerhaave and Sydenham were Redman's two principal guides in theory and practice.[22] It is perhaps significant that he presented a copy of the works of each to the library of the College of Physicians. Their doctrine, which put the patient at the center of every medical situation, appealed to Redman's personal humanity; he shared their practical good sense, and, like them, accepted truth where he found it. His master John Kearsley had once found the hint for a successful treatment in an old author. "And may not this be a hint also to us," Redman asked his brethren in the College of Physicians,

not to slight or neglect the practical observations of even antiquated authors, because they do not quadrate with the more enlightened theories of the present day? Yea, tho' we may with some reason . . . smile at their mode of theorizing upon them, let us rather . . . give them all the credit we can, for their great and often painful attention to what might conduce to the progress of the healing art and the benefit of mankind; and but for which possibly we might not have yet been so far advanced in successful

19 Benjamin Waterhouse to Redman, Dec. 20, 1790, Manuscript Archives, 145, College of Physicians.

20 Redman to Rush, Apr. 4, 1767, Rush Manuscripts, XXII, 10.

21 Redman to Rush, Dec. 21, 1782, Jan. 1, 1793, Jan. 5, 1802, *ibid.*, XXII, 21, 13, 17.

22 [Rush], "Memoirs," *Philadelphia Medical Museum*, V (1808), [51]-[52]. Mrs. Grace Growden Galloway, a friend and patient of Redman's, sketched a different picture. Ill, she sent two calls to Redman, "but he made excuses & wou'd not come." Next day, when he did visit her, he displayed "such Contempt & disregard that I wish I had not sent for him—he wou'd scarce hear what I had to say." But Mrs. Galloway, whose husband was a refugee under British protection and whose property in Philadelphia was threatened with confiscation, was overwrought at this time. Raymond C. Werner, ed., "Diary of Grace Growden Galloway," *PMHB*, LV (1931), 81.

practice as we now are, whatever we might have been in diversity of theories. Is not old Sydenham an eminent instance of the truth of the above observation?[23]

This moderate therapeutic practice, according to Rush, Redman subsequently modified. When William Cullen and John Brown called some of Boerhaave's doctrines into question, Redman considered their arguments and adopted some of their views and methods. Still later he asked to read Rush's "whole Course [of lectures on medicine] regularly thro' " for they pleased him "much."[24] Redman, Rush asserted in the obituary of his old preceptor, "considered a greater *force* of medicine necessary to cure modern American, than modern British diseases, and hence he was a decided friend to depletion in all the violent diseases of our country." These views Redman held, if he ever held them, at the end of his life. While he was one of Philadelphia's busiest doctors he practiced Hippocratic medicine. In the yellow fever of 1762, for example, he used saline purgatives successfully; in the more widespread epidemic of 1793 he still seemed to prefer them to bleeding and heroic doses of calomel and jalap.

Like all good doctors, Redman appreciated the patient's mental state as an important condition of successful treatment. In the sick room, Rush remembered, Redman "suspended pain by his soothing manner, or chased it away by his conversation," which was grave or gay, instructive or anecdotal, as the nature of the patient's illness and psychological condition indicated. A woman whom he attended during a fatal sickness told one of her friends that death had nothing terrible in it when Dr. Redman spoke to her about it. (S. Weir Mitchell a century later envied Redman the secret of his "anaesthetic kindness."[25]) When his patients kept well, Redman visited them two or three times a year all the same. Treating female patients, like Mrs. Elizabeth Graeme Ferguson, for example, he not only prescribed medicines, but often also wrote them letters, paid them visits which seemed merely social, counseled them on personal and business affairs quite unconnected with health and disease. "By no

---

[23] Redman, *An Account of The Yellow Fever as it prevailed in Philadelphia in the Autumn of 1762* . . . (Philadelphia, 1865), 39–40. The original manuscript is in the College of Physicians.

[24] Redman to Rush, Jan. 1, 1793, Rush Manuscripts, XXII, 13.

[25] S. Weir Mitchell, "Commemorative Address," College of Physicians, *Transactions*, 3rd Series, IX (1887), cccxlv.

means" should Mrs. Ferguson sell the mansion house, he advised strongly in 1782, "and . . . you ought to keep two hundred acres with it."[26]

Redman's practice, like his whole view of life, was deeply influenced by an invincible religious faith. If Redman's appreciation of the moral causes of physical effects made him aware that the strongest medication may sometimes prove useless, his Christian conviction that God has ordained all things made him cautious in initiating radical treatments or claiming credit for their cures.

John Redman's name first appears on the rolls of the Second Presbyterian Church in Philadelphia in 1744 as *juvenis*—a young man. Soon after he established himself permanently in the city, he assumed increased responsibilities for the temporal work of the church. He was a member of the committee of the congregation after 1760, a member of the committee appointed in 1761 "to wait on Robert Smith Carpenter for a plan for the Steeple," one of the collectors of pew rent. On one occasion, "Application being made by Mr. Matthew Clarkson to the Committee to remove Mrs. Clymer & Betsey Roberdeau from his seat in the church, which they have no right to & refuse to give up to him—the Committee therefore requests Dr. Redman to speak to those ladies & entreat them to give up. . . ." Redman accordingly waited on the trespassing females and the matter was happily adjusted. When the Second Church was incorporated, Redman was elected a trustee; he was subsequently vice-president, and, from 1786 to 1803, served as president of the Consistory.[27] He became an elder in 1784, for many years made an annual gift for the relief of poor women of the church, and was a constant reader of devotional literature.[28] In this his taste ran to piety rather than disputations or dogmatic theology; he hailed the popular evangelical preacher and writer Elhanan Winchester, for example, a Baptist with Universalist leanings, as "our *Theological Newton*."[29]

26 See, for example, the letters of Redman to Mrs. Ferguson, May 3, 1773, June 6, 1776, Feb. 26, 1782, in HSP. Other data on Redman's practice may be found in Drinker, 95 *et passim*.

27 Second Presbyterian Church, Congregational Minutes, I, *passim*; Minutes of the Corporation, I, II, *passim*, typescripts in Presbyterian Historical Society, Philadelphia.

28 Second Presbyterian Church, Consistory Book, 1744/5–1798, *passim*, typescript, Presbyterian Historical Society; Isaac Snowden *et al.* to Ashbel Green, Dec. 25, 1793, HSP.

29 Rush to Elhanan Winchester, Nov. 12, 1791, Butterfield, I, 611.

Such constant service to the church and contemplation of religious purposes through half a century was at once an expression of, and a stimulus to, his faith. When the church's minister Ashbel Green, vacationing in Princeton in September, 1797, debated whether to return to Philadelphia, where yellow fever was raging, Redman addressed him not as a physician but as a fellow Christian.

Mr. Falconer & myself still continue to conceive it to be your duty to venture, and beside other reasons offerd to yourself before, we think that if it be deemed improper or unjustifiable for medical doctors, & natural parents to quit us at such times, it is equally if not more so, for our spiritual fathers to desert us alltogether, or at least not occasionally to aid the remainder of their flock who cannot, or dare not emigrate, in their worship, & improvement on the present calomitous occasion. Nevertheless we do not pretend to dictate, much less to censure others, but leave them to judge for themselves, withall praying spiritual light, & supernal direction & strength may be afforded them therein.[30]

Like an ancient Christian John Redman looked forward to death. Doubtless the poor state of his health from middle age onward made him constantly aware of bodily weakness and the uncertainties of life. But there was nothing gloomy in his looking on "that Grim old *Gentleman*," as he once called death. On the contrary, he spoke of it, Rush declared, as other men speak of going to bed or journeying to a pleasant, distant country.

This stalwart Christian faith had some clearly definable effects on Redman's medical practice. Quite as much as his Hippocratic good sense, this seems to explain Redman's constant reminders to his students and colleagues that God rules and overrules the physician. He was skeptical of systems and theories, was no enthusiast for general reforms, not only because, as a man of science, he was conscious of the limitations of human knowledge, but because, as a Christian, he believed that God in his providence has decreed life and death, pain, suffering and health for each man. When Rush wrote him excitedly of the expansive ideas he was getting from his Edinburgh teachers, Redman reminded the young man that "however pleasing the prospect may be of returning to our friends fill'd with knowledge and qualified to be usefull, it is only a possession of the one thing needfull, that can make us happy in ourselves, a real

30 Redman to Ashbel Green, Sept. 20, 1797, HSP.

blessing in our generation . . . ," and that "one thing needfull," in Redman's view, was not knowledge of medicine but faith in God.[31] Similarly, when John Morgan proposed, in the interest of raising the standards of practice in this country and perhaps of carrying on some physiological researches, to practice medicine but not surgery and to sell no drugs, Redman addressed him a little sermon on Christian charity, clearly implying that a physician ought to "be every hour engaged in doing good to rich & poor, relieving the distresses of poor suffering fellow mortals, and perhaps receiving daily blessings of those who are ready to perish. . . . No life can be happy or pleasing to God but what is usefull to man."[32] And he expressed like ideas in his inaugural address as president of the College of Physicians in 1787.[33]

As he withdrew from practice and turned his mind increasingly to religious contemplations Redman seems almost to have come to accept disease as a part of the order of the universe, which it verged on impiety to alter. "The yellow fever," Redman told Mrs. Elizabeth Drinker quietly in 1798, "is progressing, and will progress; 'tis according to the nature of things at this season of the year," and he talked of going with his wife and daughter to the country.[34] When Mrs. Redman, his "Fellow Traveller in the thorny mazes of time," became ill, he half apologized for asking Rush to visit her.

And though I hope the sickness is not unto death but for the glory of God; yet after a union of thirty years, the most distant prospect of a

31 Redman to Rush, Apr. 4, 1767, Rush Manuscripts, XXII, 10.

32 Redman to [John Morgan], Mar. 13, 1764, draft, Gilbert Collection of Manuscript Letters, III, 354, College of Physicians.

33 Ruschenberger, 179–183.

34 Drinker, 133; Redman to Ashbel Green, Nov. 5, 1793, Mitchell Collection, HSP; Redman to Green, Sept. 14, 1798, College of Physicians. Redman's wife was Mary Sobers, born 1724. They had two sons, who died young, and two daughters. Anne lived with her parents until her death in 1806. Sarah married Daniel Coxe, a member of the Governor's Council of New Jersey, who was a Loyalist in the Revolution; she joined him in England in 1785. Their son, John Redman Coxe, returned to Philadelphia, where he received his medical education and had a long and distinguished career. In 1807, Sarah Redman Coxe returned to Philadelphia to visit her aged parents. They eagerly awaited her coming, Redman assuring Benjamin Rush that he "owed ten thousand talents for this new debt contracted to Heaven." Mrs. Redman survived her daughter's arrival only two months; she died Nov. 29, 1807. The doctor followed a few months later, dying from a stroke on Mar. 19, 1808. Mrs. Coxe returned to England in 1810. Rush, Autobiography, 272, 314; Redman to Rush, June 25, [1785], Rush Manuscripts, XXII, 20; Mary Redman to Elizabeth Graeme Ferguson, [June 6, 1776], HSP; Rush to Ashbel Green, June 2, 1810, PMHB, LXXII (1948), 274; Poulson's Daily American Advertiser, Mar. 23, 1808.

separation . . . makes one shudder, especially in the present circumstances. And though to depart hence and be with Christ I know would be far better for her, but to remain longer here . . . I hope would be better for me;. nevertheless . . . as all prudent means are rational . . . a visit from you will be very acceptable, and much oblige your old (paternal) friend.[35]

Another medical consequence of his Christian resignation was to discourage any inclination Redman might have had to carry out systematic observations or investigations into medicine. He wrote a defense of inoculation, which was printed in the *Pennsylvania Gazette*, July 3, 1760. His paper on the yellow fever of 1762, written at the time of the disastrous plague of 1793, was not a systematic study, but a collection of observations, an account of the treatments the doctors tried, based on his old daybook and the recollections of "an ancient woman and others" whom Redman remembered he had attended.[36] Redman was, in short, as Benjamin Smith Barton complained, one of "the *large* number of those practitioners of the healing art, who mix, for years, with the sick, and who scarcely leave behind them one important memorandum of what they have observed, in regard to the nature of diseases, or the effects, whether good or bad, of medicines." The capacity for making accurate observations, Barton conceded, was not common, even among physicians. "But every physician, possessed of a good understanding, has it in his power to augment the mass of MEDICAL FACTS, and thereby to extend the certainty and usefulness of the most important of all sciences."[37]

John Redman was the first president of the College of Physicians of Philadelphia in 1786. He was not the founder of this medical society—the College was the work of others—and though he was one of the oldest Fellows, he was not the most famous. The names of Morgan, Shippen, and Rush were better and more widely known, but none of these men could have been elected head of a Philadelphia medical society without dividing it at its birth. Redman, on the contrary, a successful practitioner, wise and tolerant, was held in esteem by all. He was re-elected president annually until, at his own request, he was allowed to retire in 1804.[38]

35 Redman to Rush, Feb. 25, 1782, Rush Manuscripts, XXII, 12.

36 John H. Powell, *Bring Out Your Dead* (Philadelphia, 1949), 87–89.

37 *Philadelphia Medical and Physical Journal*, III, Pt. 1 (1808), 189–190.

38 Redman to Vice-President and Members of the College of Physicians, July 2, 1804, Manuscript Archives, 429, College of Physicians; Redman to Thomas Mifflin, Sept. 26, 1799, HSP; Drinker, 127.

As president of the College Redman reigned rather than ruled. He presided at regular meetings when he was well enough to attend; he called special meetings when the Fellows petitioned for them or the governor of the Commonwealth requested one; he received communications addressed to him as president, passed them over to the secretary to answer, and signed the replies when they were drafted. He rejoiced publicly that the vice-presidents of the College during these years were younger men and vigorous.[39]

One is left to wonder what the source of his reputation was; why, for example, despite his repeated absences and his constant disclaimers of capacity, the physicians of Philadelphia elected him president of the College year after year. What made him by common assent the Nestor of the medical profession in Philadelphia?

In the first place, John Redman was an able physician, the teacher of able men—Morgan, Rush, and Caspar Wistar, Ralph Assheton, Samuel Treat, and Isaac Cathrall—and he was devoted to his profession. Rush preserved a toast which Redman proposed on some occasion:

> The dignity & success of the healing art.—And long health, competent wealth & exquisite happiness
> To the individual practitioner, who makes the health, comfort & happiness of his fellow mortall one of the chief ends & delights of his life; and acts therein from motives that render him superior to all difficulties he may have to encounter in the pursuit thereof.[40]

The man who can offer that toast *is* at the head of his profession.

Another reason for Redman's reputation has been suggested by W. B. McDaniel, II. Redman may have owed "the robes, at least, of power" to the "sedulously cultivated image of himself as an aged and infirm patriarch." From the time he was forty John Redman spoke constantly in his letters of his age, his weakness, his sickness, pain, and forgetfulness in tones which could only produce concern, sympathy, and even love.[41] The physicians were not alone in reacting as

39 Redman, Address on his re-election as president, 1791, Manuscript Archives, 393, College of Physicians.

40 "Dr. Redman's Toast," Rush Manuscripts, XXII, 8.

41 W. B. McDaniel, II, " 'Your Aged Friend and Fellow Servant, John Redman,' " College of Physicians, *Transactions & Studies*, 4th Series, IX (1941), 35–41. Someone, possibly Rush, in a letter, Aug. 23, 1782, reminded Redman that he should count his blessings, that he had escaped all kinds of early death, had health and reason, reputation and prosperity. *Evangelical Intelligencer*, n.s., II (1808), 326–329.

Mr. McDaniel has suggested they may have—the trustees of the Second Presbyterian Church treated Redman in the same way, possibly for the same reason.

Finally, of course, Redman's contemporaries respected him because he was so patently a man of integrity and good will. His manners were antique; a new generation of physicians, taught by Rush, thought him too cautious in practice; and his gaze was too steadily fixed on heaven to make him an apt ally of those who were doing the world's work in Philadelphia.[42] But there was nothing grasping, proud, or contentious about Redman. Only goodness came from him even as a young man, for if his temper overcame him and he spoke sharply to an apprentice, he never failed to apologize promptly; and as an old man, unlike others of his class and generation, he praised Thomas Paine and thought it "strange . . . & wonderfull, that even the madness . . . of the people in France, should be made the means of accomplishing the grand purpose of their own liberation, liberty, & political happiness, probably sooner, & possibly much firmer than would have been done by the exercise of their sober reason & senses. . . ."[43]

The one humorous anecdote told of him seems out of character, seems in fact as though it should have been told of Abraham Chovet: that when a stranger importuned him in a public place for advice about a pain in the chest, Redman replied, after a solemn pause, that his advice in the case was that the patient—consult his doctor. In an age of loud, contentious Hippocrats, he was remarkable for sound sense, humility, charity, and quiet confidence. For these qualities Redman was respected by all and liked by many; and most men cheerfully allowed him the title he had assumed with modest but affectionate pride in 1787—that of the professional father of the physicians of Philadelphia.

---

[42] Redman's general civic activity was solid and unspectacular. He was a trustee of the College of Philadelphia, 1751–1791, and of Princeton, 1761–1778. He was a member of the American Philosophical Society, the Agricultural Society, and the Prison Society of Philadelphia, but in none of these was he as active as in the Consistory of his church.

[43] Redman to Rush, Jan. 1, 1793, Rush Manuscripts, XXII, 13.

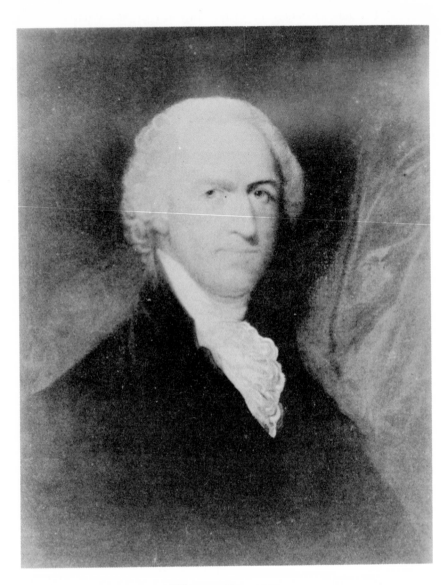

WILLIAM SHIPPEN

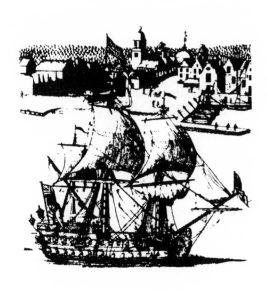

Philadelphia Medical Students in Europe, 1750–1800

ORE than half the twenty-four founding members of the College of Physicians of Philadelphia in 1787 had received a part of their formal medical training in Europe; and when in the succeeding decade Caspar Wistar, Junior, Benjamin Smith Barton, Philip Syng Physick, and Isaac Cathrall began to practice, the number of Philadelphia physicians with foreign education was increased. What was true of Quakerdelphia was true also, though usually to a lesser degree, elsewhere in the United States. From 1749, when John Moultrie, of South Carolina, was made a doctor of medicine of the University of Edinburgh, to the close of the century, no fewer than 117 Americans received the medical degree of that institution alone; while uncounted others, like Thomas Parke, Samuel Powel Griffitts, and Benjamin Smith Barton, studied there for a term or two. Indeed, so constant was the flow of American medical students to England, Scotland, and the Continent in the latter half of the eighteenth century, that one might speak of a kind of trade in them, America exporting the raw materials for physicians

and surgeons and receiving after the passage of three or four years
the finished products. These colonials and young republicans filled
themselves at the fountainheads of science abroad; and, returning
with the knowledge of the European schools and hospitals, were prepared and eager, the Philadelphians at least, to spread their learning
through the United States and make Philadelphia the Edinburgh of
America.[1]

The medical students who went abroad in the half century after
1750 were not, however, pioneers in a new movement, for in the
second quarter of the century several Philadelphians had sought
medical instruction in England and on the Continent. John Redman
and Benjamin Morris received their degrees from Leyden; Thomas
Bond studied in Paris and Thomas Cadwalader in London with
Cheselden and at Rheims; and at Rheims Phineas Bond received his
medical degree.[2] These were the men who dominated the profession
in the city at mid-century and were the preceptors of that group of
younger men who made Philadelphia at the century's close the
medical capital of the nation. These older men, who, like Redman,
could speak of many of the members of the College of Physicians as
their professional children, established a standard of medical practice
and fashioned a pattern of professional education which no prospective student of medicine, especially if he wished to practice in
Philadelphia, could safely ignore.

Drawn to the practice of medicine for varying reasons—Wistar is
said to have been moved by the suffering of the wounded at the

---

1 Any study of this subject must begin by owning its indebtedness to Francis R. Packard,
"How London and Edinburgh Influenced Medicine in Philadelphia in the Eighteenth Cen-
tury," *Annals of Medical History*, n.s., IV (1932), 219–44; to Dr. Packard's *History of Medicine
in the United States* (New York, 1931), II, 951ff; to J. Gordon Wilson, "The Influence of
Edinburgh on American Medicine in the 18th Century," Institute of Medicine of Chicago,
Proceedings, VII (1929), 129–38; to Michael Kraus, "American and European Medicine in
the Eighteenth Century," *Bulletin of the History of Medicine*, VIII (1940), 679–95; and to
William S. Middleton's sketches of the lives of eminent Philadelphia physicians of the eighteenth century which have appeared from time to time in the *Annals of Medical History*.

2 It is not easy to determine the nature of the foreign studies of some of these men and
their successors. Within their limits the following lists are helpful: R. W. Innes Smith,
English-Speaking Students of Medicine at the University of Leyden (Edinburgh, 1932) and *List
of the Graduates in Medicine in the University of Edinburgh, from MDCCV. to MDCCCLXVI.*
(Edinburgh, 1867), from the last of which Samuel Lewis extracted the names of the American
students, which were printed in the *New England Historical and Genealogical Register*, XLII
(1888), 159–65.

battle of Germantown,[3] while Barton may have studied physic to give respectability to his study of botany and natural history—these young men entered upon a course of study already pretty well fixed for them. The best preparation was a college education, then three or more years of apprenticeship to a learned and reputable physician, and finally Europe for what William Shippen, Junior, called "the last polish." Shippen himself followed this program—a bachelor's degree at the College of New Jersey, three years' study with his father in Philadelphia, and then anatomical studies in London, the medical degree at Edinburgh, and a visit to Paris. John Morgan and Benjamin Rush also received their medical training in these three stages, as did John Carson, Philip Syng Physick, and Thomas T. Hewson,[4] the last three all graduates of the college at Philadelphia. But John Morgan's dream of basing medical studies on a broad liberal education failed to materialize even in his own school; probably the greater number entered upon their apprenticeship and medical studies without having been to college and, receiving the degree of bachelor of medicine, either set up in practice at once or went abroad to receive the coveted M.D. in Scotland or on the Continent. To this group belonged Thomas Parke, who, however, was content not to take his degree, Caspar Wistar, Junior, James Hutchinson, Samuel Powel Griffitts, and John Foulke. John Redman Coxe probably belongs in their number as well, for after he received his M.D. from the University of Pennsylvania (the degree of bachelor of medicine was dropped in 1789), he spent one year in the London Hospital and another attending the lectures and hospitals at Edinburgh and Paris.[5] Only Thomas Ruston seems to have gone to Europe directly from his apprenticeship without a formal liberal or medical education.[6] But none went to Europe without an apprenticeship of some sort. So important indeed was this element of training that when George Logan arrived in London without it, Dr. Fothergill

---

[3] William S. Middleton, "Caspar Wistar, Junior," *Annals of Medical History*, IV (1922), 64.

[4] Franklin Bache, *An Obituary Notice of Thomas T. Hewson, M.D.,* . . . (Phila., 1850), 3-4. Hewson was the son of that William Hewson, F.R.S., pupil and assistant of the Hunters, with whom some of the Philadelphia medical students worked in London.

[5] Mary Clapier Coxe, "A Biographical Sketch of John Redman Coxe, M.D., and John Redman, M.D.," *University of Pennsylvania Medical Bulletin*, XX (1908), 294-95.

[6] James Pemberton to John Fothergill, [Philadelphia] 6 mo. 3, 1763. Pemberton Papers (Historical Society of Pennsylvania), XXXIV, 153.

sent him off at once to spend a year studying and working with a country practitioner.[7]

What a medical student learned from his apprenticeship depended, naturally, upon the character of his preceptor and the nature of the work he was required and permitted to do. The labors of an apprentice ran the gamut from errand boy to physician-in-charge: Rush, for example, after only a year's observation and practice, was frequently left by Dr. Redman in full charge of a patient.[8] Once when Logan and his preceptor differed as to the cause of death from a blow, the latter requested and received permission for the two of them to examine the body.[9] Such practical training as this was, of course, based upon a study of the medical masters: Rush learned his Hippocrates by translating the *Aphorisms* into English;[10] and Dr. Kuhn, putting young Physick through a thorough course of reading, directed him first of all to master Cullen's *First Lines*, an injunction the boy obeyed by memorizing the entire work.[11] And from the manuscript notes of the lectures of the teachers in London and Edinburgh, which appear to have circulated among the medical students in Philadelphia, the students received an introduction to the latest medical and allied doctrines and a preparation for their own attendance upon the same or similar lectures.

But here the resources of Philadelphia ended. To an English correspondent the elder Dr. Shippen wrote, "My son has had his education in the best college in this part of the country, and has been studying physic with me, besides which he has had the opportunity of seeing the practice of every gentleman of note in our city. But for want of that variety of operations and those frequent dissections which are common in older countries, I must send him to Europe." There the younger Shippen might spend a winter in London, attending William Hunter's anatomical lectures and private dissections, take a course in midwifery with Smellie, and enter himself as a pupil at Guy's Hospital; then he might go on to Rouen, study physic and take his degree; and finally he might return to London and revisit

7 Logan to Charles Logan, Dunmow, Aug. 16, 1775. Letter Book (H S P).

8 Nathan G. Goodman, *Benjamin Rush, Physician and Citizen, 1746–1813* (Phila., 1934), 10.

9 Logan to Charles Logan, Dunmow, March, 1776. Letter Book (H S P).

10 Goodman, *op. cit.*, 11.

11 Charles Caldwell, *A Discourse Commemorative of Philip Syng Physick, M.D.* . . . . (Louisville, Ky., 1838), 9.

the hospitals.[12] Such a letter might have been written and such a program outlined for any one of a dozen Philadelphia medical students.

When his American education was completed, therefore, his resolve taken to go abroad, and his passage booked, the medical student turned to his Philadelphia instructors for letters of introduction to the great and near-great of the medical and scientific worlds of Britain and the Continent which he was about to enter. Benjamin Franklin, Dr. Fothergill and Dr. Lettsom, London physicians, the Barclays, great men in the Quaker hierarchy, and other friends of Americans received a constant stream of young Philadelphians—Franklin's "American children," Thomas Bond called them[13]—bearing letters from America; and in their turn they provided the young men with other letters which might be useful to them in the prosecution of their studies. Fothergill never failed to receive an American, and especially a Pennsylvania Quaker, with grave courtesy and Friendly kindness. He made him welcome, and proposed a course of study. Logan, for example, he received "in such manner as had more the appearance of a tender Father than a transient Friend."[14] Franklin introduced the students to persons of his acquaintance, advised them on their studies and bearing, sometimes even loaned them money. He gave Rush, when Rush set out for France, a letter of credit on a Paris banker;[15] and he loaned John Morgan the amount of the fees involved in that Philadelphian's election to the Royal Society of London.[16]

A few, asking for more than letters of introduction, requested advice on the proper course of study and conduct abroad. For John Foulke, who sailed to France in the spring of 1780, and for Samuel Powel Griffitts, who went over the next year, Dr. Rush prepared a list of eighteen suggestions. Evincing not only a care for the profes-

[12] Packard, *History of Medicine in the United States*, II, 970, quoting John F. Watson, *Annals of Philadelphia* . . . (Phila. 1844), II, 378.

[13] Bond to Benjamin Franklin, Philadelphia, April 27, 1780. Franklin Papers (American Philosophical Society), XVIII, 49.

[14] Logan to Charles Logan, London, July 10, 1775. Letter Book (H S P).

[15] Goodman, *op. cit.*, 19.

[16] Morgan to Franklin, Philadelphia, Oct. 10, 1765. Franklin Papers (A P S), I, 162. There is an interesting exchange of letters between Rush and Jonathan Potts and Dr. Franklin in Mrs. Thomas Potts James, *Memorial of Thomas Potts, Junior* . . . (Privately printed, 1874), 172–75.

sional advancement of his students, but an interest in their social development as well, Rush recommended that Foulke and Griffitts attend lectures on natural philosophy as well as on medical subjects, visit the hospitals, noting the prescriptions and modes of treatment, spend a few hours daily for some weeks in a chemical laboratory and apothecary's shop, and acquire a library. He also urged them to keep a diary, "Attend Shews of all kinds, and describe in your Journal"— this a reflection of Rush's own stern morality—"the most trifling of them," and spend an hour daily for three months in dancing lessons.[17] Indeed, the ease and success with which the Americans made their way in the scientific and social world of Europe was a tribute not only to their knowledge, intelligence, and lively interest, but to their social grace and personal charm as well.[18]

In addition to letters of introduction and advice, those Philadelphians who were also Friends usually wished to take with them a certificate from their meeting. Probably typical was that issued to Charles Moore, who went to Edinburgh in 1748, which certified that he was "Religiously disposed . . . a diligent Attender of our Meetings for Worship & . . . clear from Marriage Engagements."[19] Caspar Wistar, when he applied for a similar certificate, had some difficulty in obtaining it, for Wistar the preceding fall had fallen "into the Scandalous & alarming temptation of being engaged in a duel"; and though he had publicly condemned his conduct, the elders of the meeting inclined to feel that he ought to evidence in his outward port a greater proof of humiliation and contrition of heart.[20] That Friends were not without grounds for their fear of the temptations which might befall those removed from the oversight of the meeting is attested by the cases of Jonas Preston and Samuel Powel

[17] Rush, "Letters, Facts & Observations upon a Variety of Subjects," 47–51. Rush MSS. (Library Company of Philadelphia, Ridgway Branch). Dr. Rush had followed his own advice in the matter of a journal. The journal of his studies at Edinburgh and London, 1766–68, has recently come to light and is now (October, 1942) in the possession of Mr. James Lewis Hook, a dealer in early Americana, of Bala-Cynwyd, Pa. The journal of Rush's European tour is owned by the Pierpont Morgan Library, New York City, but, being in safe-keeping for the duration, could not be consulted in the preparation of this paper.

[18] William Cullen to Rush, Edinburgh, Aug. 16, 1785. Rush MSS. (L C P, Ridgway), XXIV, 58.

[19] Pennsylvania Magazine of History and Biography, XVII (1893), 379.

[20] James Pemberton to John Pemberton, Philadelphia, 8 mo. 27, 1783. Pemberton Papers (H S P), XXXIX, 89.

Griffitts. The first, when he reached Paris, adopted an extreme manner of Parisian dress and speech, to the great concern of his mother, a respected preacher among Friends;[21] while the latter hardly set foot on French soil than he returned to his mother his inexpensive American watch "as it would make but a poor Appearance here, where we cannot expect People to value such Things for their intrinsic Worth."[22] Still, as he was resolved to go to Edinburgh in any case, Wistar got his certificate and departed with the blessing, albeit reluctant, of the meeting.

No medical student set out for Europe without having first considered with his preceptor and medical school instructors at Philadelphia the advantages of the several schools abroad. Dr. Thomas Bond, one of the sanest of the Philadelphia physicians, when he was inquiring after a proper school for his son Richard, made a rapid survey of them in 1771. "The School of Edinburgh," he began, "seems at this time to be better calculated to please the Fancy, than to form the Judgement; and indeed the many extraordinary Novelties incullcated there, would be a Barr to public Confidence in this Part of the World. As far as We can judge from the public Exhibitions," he went on, "Surgery in London is a *mere mechanic* Art, well executed." Of Paris he could make no judgment, for his friends and former teachers there, Astruc, Winslow, Ferin, Huno, and Le Cat, were all dead. He reckoned that if the writings of Gaubius were any criterion, physic must be scientifically and usefully taught at Leyden, though the school was said to be neglected. The medical institutions of Vienna he knew had been reformed by Van Swieten, which was good; yet the world was annually misled by absurdities and falsehoods propagated under his sanctions, this was bad.[23] But in spite of Bond's judgment of Edinburgh, "the general Run" of students from America, as Dr. Franklin put it, was to the Scottish capital.[24] Naturally the language barrier tended to deflect the stream from the Continent, while tradition, common citizenship, the advice of Fother-

21 Richard C. Norris, "The Preston Retreat," in Frederick P. Henry, editor, *Founders' Week Memorial Volume* (Phila., 1909), 781–82.

22 Griffitts to Abigail Griffitts, L'Orient, Sept. 9, 1781. Griffitts Correspondence (H S P).

23 Bond to Franklin, Philadelphia, July 6, 1771, in William Pepper, "The Medical Side of Benjamin Franklin," *University of Pennsylvania Medical Bulletin*, XXIII (1910), 333–35.

24 Franklin to Bond, London, Feb. 5, 1772, in Pepper, "The Medical Side of Benjamin Franklin," *loc. cit.*, 336–39.

gill and Lettsom, both Edinburgh graduates, and the dazzling eminence of Edinburgh itself all strengthened the pull to that center. Nothing less than war, in fact, was able to break the Philadelphia-Edinburgh-London pattern of medical education. During the American Revolution Foulke and Griffitts studied at Paris. The former went on to Leipsic and the latter, considering physic "not on so respectable a Footing" in Paris as one might wish, to Montpellier.[25] But both, as soon as returning peace permitted them to enter England, made straight for the teachers of their American teachers. None ever ventured as far as Vienna. However, Hugh Williamson, after studies at Edinburgh, London, and Leyden, took his degree at Utrecht in 1766,[26] and Barton, piqued at some real or fancied indifference on the part of two of the faculty, left Edinburgh for Germany, where he is said—though a search of the records failed to reveal the truth of the allegation—to have received his medical degree at Göttingen.[27] And although Morgan made a well-known visit to Padua, he seems to have carried away from his interviews with the aged Morgagni only the two stout volumes of a presentation copy of the *De Sedibus et Causis Morborum*,[28] and none followed his steps below the Alps.

So for the Philadelphia medical student it was pretty largely a story of Edinburgh and London.[29] Boerhaave's Scottish students, returned from Leyden, had made the Scottish capital a live and throbbing center of medical teaching, the most famous certainly and the most influential in the latter half of the eighteenth century. In

25 Griffitts to Rush, Paris, Sept. 19, 1782. Rush MSS. (L C P, Ridgway), XLIII, 73.

26 David Hosack, *A Biographical Memoir of Hugh Williamson, M.D., LL. D.* (New York, 1821), 18–19.

27 Edgar Fahs Smith, *Benjamin Smith Barton: An American Naturalist* ([Phila.] 1916), 10; William P. C. Barton, *A Biographical Sketch . . . of . . . Professor Barton* (n.p. [1816]), 12–13.

28 John Morgan, *Journal . . . from the City of Rome to the City of London, 1764 . . .* (Phila., 1907), 104–108; Richard H. Shryock, "The Advent of Modern Medicine in Philadelphia, 1800–1850," *Yale Journal of Biology and Medicine*, XIII (1941), 724. My indebtedness to Professor Shryock is far greater than is indicated by this single citation.

29 For a general picture of Edinburgh in the last third of the century, see the pleasant chapters, especially the last, "Edinburgh in Robertson's Time," in John Harrison, *Oure Tounis Colledge: Sketches of the History of the Old College of Edinburgh* (Edinburgh, 1884). A fine description of the medical school, student life, the organization of medical instruction, and the opportunities of medical education, is presented by D. M. Lyon, "A Student of 1765–70—A Glimpse of Eighteenth Century Medicine," *Edinburgh Medical Journal*, XLVIII (1941), 185–208, an article based on letters of John Ravenscroft, of Virginia.

the 1780s nearly five hundred students of medicine were in the city—
John R. B. Rodgers in the spring of 1785 said that Dr. Monro had
399 in his anatomy class alone[30]—and of this number there were
always fifteen or twenty Americans, usually two or three Philadelphians. Most of the students were younger than those from the
Quaker City and not so well prepared, for they came straight to
Edinburgh to serve their apprenticeship and attend the lectures
together; and many were so rude and boisterous that Wistar distinguished from the throng those whom he called "respectable."[31] In
fact one medical student from Virginia, looking back on his life at
Edinburgh, expressed the opinion that "more licentious youths are
hardly to be found anywhere than I remember to have seen in
Edinburgh." Another from the Old Dominion in 1776 divided the
students into three groups: "the Fine Gentlemen," who did not
study; "the Gentlemen, or students of medicine strictly speaking,"
who lived genteely yet applied themselves to their work; and "the
vulgar," who were either lazy or "entirely devoid of everything
polite and agreeable."[32]

The Philadelphians seem to have belonged almost without exception in the number of "the Gentlemen, or students of medicine
strictly speaking." Most of them had had some formal medical
instruction at home and all had served an apprenticeship with some
practitioner. They were, therefore, if not mature, at least older than
the common run, and they had had a certain amount of experience.
One would expect them to be, like Thomas Parke, astonished and
disgusted by "the Indecency, Ill manner & foolish Conduct of many
of the Pupils" in London at Dr. McKenzie's demonstration of the
female reproductive organs.[33] Furthermore, several of the Philadelphians, like Rush, went to Europe to prepare themselves to teach at
home; while all Americans, whether they were still colonials or were
erstwhile subjects of the Crown, felt they were on their mettle to
prove themselves by the excellence of their work.

Their mornings were largely occupied in hearing lectures read, and

[30] Rodgers to Rush, Edinburgh, April 4, 1785. Rush MSS. (L C P, Ridgway), XXV, 5.
[31] Wistar to Thomas Wistar, Edinburgh, Feb. 14, 1785. Vaux Papers (H S P).
[32] Wyndham B. Blanton, *Medicine in Virginia in the Eighteenth Century* (Richmond, Va.,
1931), 89. Pages 83–92 provide a good account of the Virginia students at Edinburgh in the
latter half of the century.
[33] Thomas Parke, Journal, No. 1, Aug. 16, 1771. Pemberton Papers (H S P), LVII, 93.

the notes taken then were written out in full in the afternoon or evening. In addition there were at Edinburgh—though this was hardly a feature of the course—some opportunities for hospital observation in the Royal Infirmary; and most of the students employed a part of their free time in reading some of the most recent professional publications. There were letters to write: nothing delighted the medical students more than to be able to detail a course of experiments or to keep their old preceptors at Philadelphia informed of the latest opinions and discoveries in the medical and scientific world. When the use of opium in the treatment of syphilis was being hotly debated in the 1780s, for example, Wistar and James Hall filled their letters to Rush with accounts of the newest developments and ventured their own careful judgments in the matter.[34] Most Americans probably belonged to one or more of the medical societies at Edinburgh. Here the opinions of the professors were examined (recorded judgments of the instructors by their students seem to suggest that those lecturers were most highly thought of who made a display of erudition and had an impressive mode of delivery) and papers were read and defended by the members. Logan, for example, read papers on dyspepsia, which he attributed to lack of exercise, on ulceration, and on small pox and inoculation.[35] Wistar was elected a president of the Royal Medical Society and of a "Society for the further Investigation of Natural History," and Logan, when he was quitting Edinburgh, wrote his brother that he did not esteem his medical degree "so great an honour as being President of the Medical Society . . . ."[36] Barton made no small splash while a student at Edinburgh. He was a president of the Royal Medical Society in 1787–88; and he won the Harveian Prize of the Society with an essay on the black henbane (*Hyoscyamus niger*). In 1787 he published his *Observations on some Parts of Natural History*, which undertook to show that the Indian mounds of North America were constructed by the Toltecs of Mexico and that the Toltecs were descended from the Danes. Although he felt this

---

34 Benjamin Smith Barton to Benjamin Rush, Edinburgh, March 21, 1787; Wistar to Rush, Edinburgh, June 26, Sept. 7, 1785; Hall to Rush, London, March 18, April 5, 1784. Rush MSS. (L C P, Ridgway), XXVII, 3; XXIX, 123, 124; XXXIII, 106; XLIII, 99.

35 Logan to Charles Logan, Edinburgh, July 5, Dec. 20, 1777, Jan. 17, 1778. Letter Book (H S P).

36 Logan to Charles Logan, Edinburgh, June 24, 1779. Letter Book (H S P).

opened up the subject, he had the good sense to regret it immediately as a "premature performance."[37]

Most of these matters concerning the medical school were touched upon in a long letter which George Logan wrote his brother from Edinburgh in 1778:[38]

The Medical department consists of 6 Professorships, Viz, Chemistry, Anatomy, Practice, Theory, Mat. Med. and Botany. These Classes every Gentleman who graduates, is obliged to attend, his attendance on Midwifery is also expected, but this they cannot insist on. You cannot graduate here without having studied Medicine at this or some other University for three years: on these conditions you are admitted to a private examination at which, if you give satisfaction you are declared a candidate; after this you have another private & one public examination; but there is hardly an instance of a Gentleman being degraded after passing his first. Your exercises consist in writing several papers for private inspection and a Thesis which you are to publish & defend at the Public examination.

D^r.s Black, Monro & Cullen who fill the three first chairs, are Men of great abilities and eminent in their different departments—Black is esteemed one of the first Chemists in Europe—he has made several discoveries with respect to fixed air, & has some peculiar Ideas respecting *latent-heat;* but unfortunate for himself & for Mankind, he allows others to publish his discoveries in an imperfect state, for which they reap the laurels only due to himself. His Lectures are more calculated for the Physician as a Philosopher than as a practitioner. D^r. Monro has generally above 300 Pupils; for as his Lectures are on Anatomy & Surgery it is necessary for persons in every department of Medicine to attend him. He is too great a Philosopher to enter so minutely into his subject as the demonstrative part of it requires, on which account Students may attend him three or four years without gaining a proper knowledge of this kind; but in his Physiology, perhaps no person is equal to him for perspicuity and strength of argument—A large fortune has lulled his genius asleep, he therefore does not fatigue himself in making new discoveries, but contents himself in delivering his Lectures nearly verbatim as he did 15 years ago.

The World is so well acquainted with D^r. Cullen's abilities that it is unnecessary to say anything with respect to them. You know he has established a new theory of Medicine; but like all other Great Men, I am afraid he is too fond of this Child, to make it of long continuance. As the Boerhaavians accounted for every disease of the body from a vitiated state of the fluids, so on the other hand D^r. Cullen refers them to a vitiated state of the Nervous System. Both these opinions have their merits & demerits; wherefore it is necessary for a student to attend several Universities, and not too early to form his opinion. . . .

The fee to each of the Professors is three Guineas except to D^r. Hope who is only allowed two by the University, yet such is his meanness that he will take three guineas not only the first but the second year if any Gentleman should do him that honour to attend him.

[37] Barton, *op. cit.,* 10–12; Alan Thomson, Librarian of the Royal Medical Society, to author, Edinburgh, Sept. 14, 1942. Mr. Thomson kindly checked the records to learn when Wistar, Barton, and Logan were elected members of the Society and when each served as president.

[38] Logan to Charles Logan, Edinburgh, March 2, 1778. Letter Book (H S P.)

The Medical Students also reap great advantage from the Infirmary to which they also pay three Guineas. It is a fine building consisting of a Body [ ] feet in length & two wings; and will contain [ ] Patients. It is regulated in a better manner than any other Hospital in Britain, but as my friend Dʳ. Stedman has lately published an account of it, I will procure one of them for you.

Another very great advantage which I have not taken notice of is derived from the 3 Medical Societies where every Member is obliged to give in Papers & defend them—Here the different doctrines & opinions of great Men are canvassed with diffidence and candor—Each Society has its own particular laws printed & Libraries to which the Members have free access—The Medical Society is the oldest established—it has a Hall not yet finished which will cost upwards of £1200 and their collection of Books is excellent & valued at £1000. I have the honor of being a Member of these three Societies from which I assure you I have received as much improvement as from any one Professor. In one of these Societies the Latin language is spoke with great fluency and ease. . . .

Among such a number of students you will no doubt judge that we have plenty of companions but I do not think that a Man of your good sense & taste would be able to select 20 out of Monro's 300 with whom you would wish to associate. On account of there being such a large proportion of the low class among the Students, the others are not paid that respect which is due to them neither from the Citizens nor Professors considering the quantity of Money they annually spend among them and their genteel behavior.

But for persons like Logan, "students of medicine strictly speaking," life in the University town was not unpleasant. They lived with private families, for Principal Robertson was no believer in student segregation as practiced in the English universities. Thus they in some measure entered into the life of the community, forming acquaintances and sometimes friendships which extended over many years. Rush, for example, was admitted as a burgess and guild brother of the city,[39] and was sufficiently at home among the Scots to persuade John Witherspoon to come to the presidency of the College of New Jersey.[40] In fact he made such intimate friends abroad that, twenty-five years later, he received a personal gift from his old friend Lady Jane Belcher.[41]

How very pleasant the life of the Philadelphians at Edinburgh might be is suggested by the experience of Thomas Parke, whom Fothergill recommended to the care of a worthy Quaker of Edinburgh, one Miller. Well known, respected, and wealthy, Friend Miller inquired assiduously into the progress of Parke and some of

39 *Notes and Queries*, IX (1854), 603. The reference was suggested by Dr. Packard and J. Gordon Wilson.

40 Goodman, *op. cit.*, 16–17.

41 Wistar to Rush, London, Aug. 14, 1786. Rush MSS. (L C P, Ridgway), XXIX, 125.

his fellow students, saw to it that they attended their religious meetings, and had them to his home each First-day evening when, after reading from the Bible or from Quaker books, with an occasional exhortation from a female preacher, they all sat down to a good supper.[42] More interesting, though less typical, of course, was the experience of Rush's fellow student, Jonathan Potts. Of Quaker inheritance, though not a birthright Friend, he had a deep religious experience on shipboard, so that when he arrived in Edinburgh he was a different man from the one who had left Philadelphia. Regularly he attended Quaker meeting in the Scottish capital. It was composed of eight or ten men and as many women, and only when some traveling Friend came was there any preaching. Hence he attended meeting for months "without ever hearing a word externally, but it has been quite otherwise inwardly . . . . I really believe," he went on, contrasting this silent meeting with the proud assemblages of the Quakers in their seat at Philadelphia, "that there is more Life & heartfelt Religion in the silent Meetings at Edinburg than in the Meetings of the highly-favored People of Phil. who have line upon line, & precept upon precept, & who perhaps overlook that indwelling Word which is not only able to direct Men to the path of Life, but will enable them to walk in it. . . ." And Potts, resolved to walk according to the Light, really humbled himself. The tickets to plays, concerts, and dances which well-meaning friends sent him had to be returned; and he was not afraid to own himself a Quaker. Off came his ruffles, his hair he untied, and he was "not ashamed to use the plain language to the greatest Man in Edinburg, not but that it is a great cross to me."[43]

As Logan wrote, Cullen was preeminent at Edinburgh, and his influence on the young students from America was stupendous. Morgan called him the Boerhaave of his age and spoke of him with emotion.[44] Thomas Parke in 1771 called him "y^t. Shining Oracle of Physic."[45] While Rush became positively ecstatic at the mention of his name: "D^r. *Cullen* the great the unrivalled D^r. *Cullen* is going on

[42] Joseph Parrish, "Biographical Notice of Dr. Thomas Parke . . .," in Biographical Sketches and Memoirs of Members of the College of Physicians of Philadelphia (MS., College of Physicians of Philadelphia), 18–19.
[43] Potts to Joseph Potts, Edinburgh, Jan. 20, 1767. Mrs. James, *op. cit.*, 177–78.
[44] Rush to Morgan, Edinburgh, Nov. 16, 1766. Gratz Collection (H S P), Case 1, Box 20.
[45] Parke, Journal, No. 2, Oct. 22, 1771. Pemberton Papers (H S P), LVII, 98.

unfolding each Day some new facet to us in the Animal Oeconomy
. . . I think I would not fail of having heard them [his lectures] for
ten thousand pounds. illustrious Oracle of human Wisdom live—
live forever!"[46] Not twenty years later another Philadelphian declared that Cullen was "certainly one of the greatest men that ever
lived—his method in arrangement & his perspicuity in argument are
astonishingly fine & convincing—like a true philosopher he makes
every thing tend to the illustration of his subject." And Rodgers
found him, as Rush had, "the Idol of his Pupils."[47] So greatly in
fact did Edinburgh and the brilliance of the Cullenian system announced there impress some of the American medical students that
they never shook free of the Scotsman's intellectual dominance.
Rush left Edinburgh in hopes that he would "be able to transplant
most of his Doctrines to Philadelphia";[48] while Kuhn's lectures at
the University of Pennsylvania were declared by the black-biled
Charles Caldwell to be a mere paraphrase of Cullen, "and not a few
of them actual copies of his lectures."[49]

Still the importance of the practical work at London was recognized. The wiser felt as Logan did: he left the northern capital
between terms to spend two months dissecting at London, "it being
a necessary & useful part of our profession, but which the prejudices
of the Scotch will not admit of our deriving any advantage from."[50]
There were some, however, who were inclined to feel that no profit
was to be derived from the hospital experience and anatomical
theaters of London by those who had received at Edinburgh the
"last polish" in medical training. This was the opinion of James
Hall, who attended John Hunter's lectures "more for the name of the
thing than anything else,"[51] and of Benjamin Rush, who began his

46 Rush to Morgan, Edinburgh, July 27, 1768. Joseph Carson, History of the Medical
Department of the University of Pennsylvania (MS. Scrapbook in College of Physicians of
Philadelphia), II, 27.

47 Rodgers to Rush, Edinburgh, July 20, 1785. Rush MSS. (L C P, Ridgway), XXV, 6;
Rush to Morgan, Edinburgh, April 27, 1768. Carson, op. cit., II, 89.

48 Rush to Morgan, Edinburgh, Jan. 20, 1768. Carson, op. cit., II, 23 (MS., College of
Physicians of Phila.).

49 Caldwell, Autobiography (Phila., 1855), 124.

50 Logan to Charles Logan, London, Sept. 6, 1777. Letter Book (H S P).

51 Hall to Rush, March 4, 1784, in W. S. W. Ruschenberger, An Account of the Institution
and Progress of the College of Physicians of Philadelphia during a Hundred Years, from January, 1787 (Phila., 1887), 17.

work in London with the conviction that he would not get "any great Improvement from it. After attending the Lectures & Practice of the great *Dr Cullen* for two years," he explained to Morgan, "I am sure little Knowledge can be acquired from the random Prescriptions of the London Hospital Physicians. however as my Reputation may be influenced by it, I shall follow them faithfully for some Months." But after a few months' experience his doubts were resolved. He conceded that the London schools had their merit and he admitted the error of his judgment of the London physicians, but with a curious reservation that shows how much he was still under the domination of system: "few of them indeed practise Medicine upon philosophical principles, but notwithstanding this, they have enriched ye Science wth. a number of very useful Facts." He was attending William Hunter's lectures and, "as soon as the Weather is cold eno' to admit of bringing dead Bodies into ye Theater," he would begin to dissect under Hewson.[52]

For it was the hospitals and the private schools that made London, as Griffitts called it, "the Metropolis of the whole World for practical Medicine";[53] and the Americans who studied in London attended the practice of the first and the lectures of the second. The usual routine called for walking the wards with a physician or surgeon, like Dr. Huck or Mr. Cline, in the morning, a lecture in the afternoon, and study, reading, or the copying of lecture notes in the evening. Occasionally there might be an operation and once in a while an invitation from one of the older men to attend a meeting of one of the medical societies. Only one criticism of the hospital work was voiced and that was the reaction against the traditional English distinction between physicians and surgeons. An American student who paid a fee to attend, say, the surgical practice of Henry Cline, was surprised and irritated to be told that if he wished to attend the prescriptions of the house physicians, he must pay the physician's fee as well. These, John Rodgers thought, were "monstrously enormous." James Hall, for example, a dresser at St.

<hr>

52 Rush to Morgan, Edinburgh, July 27, Oct. 21, 1768. Carson, *op. cit.*, II, 27, 28.

53 Griffitts to Rush, London, Aug. 10, 1783. Rush MSS. (L C P, Ridgway), XXI, 94. But Griffitts thought that the French hospitals, from which he had just come, were superior in cleanliness and nursing arrangements.

Thomas', paid £50 for the privilege. To have attended a physician would have cost him another £22, which he could not afford.[54] ·

Of equal importance with the hospitals in the London pattern of medical instruction were the schools of the private teachers of anatomy, surgery, and midwifery. The greatest names in the last third of the century were those of William and John Hunter; and some of the Philadelphians, as Shippen, Rush, Physick, Hutchinson, Wistar, Lyons, and Hall, not only attended their lectures but in some cases had the privilege of studying with them as house pupils. On October 2, 1759, William Shippen, Junior, moved his trunk to John Hunter's and began a busy period of work in the dissecting room and of attendance on William Hunter's lectures. Day after day, as his journal records, he went into the dissecting room at six or seven in the morning, worked until late afternoon, and stopped only when he must attend one of William Hunter's classes. Here are the entries of a single week:[55]

November 1. Rose at 8. busy in dissecting room all Day. Lecture at Night.

November 2. Went to Georges Hospital and saw Hawkins and Bromfield operate, Stone and amputation. Mr. Hunter in afternoon dissecting for Glands and Ducts for Saliva. Lecture at 5 till 8. New farce High Life below Stairs; very good and apropos to times.

November 3. Rose at 8. saw Mr. H. extract a Steatomatous Tumor from upper Eyelid. busy in opening a Live Dog to see the Lacteals and thoracic Duct etc. Lecture from 5 till 8.

November 4. as usual at Mr. DeBerdts.

November 5. Dissecting all Day. Lecture till 8.

November 6. looking at Mr. Hunter dissecting for Lecture the Muscles of Thigh and Leg. Lecture at 5. At Roberts till 9, sup'd and bed.

November 7. Rose at 7. Mr. Hunter dissecting Muscles for Lecture. Went to see a patient under my care. . . . After Lecture went to Bartholomews Hospital and saw the neatest operation for Bubonocele that I ever saw by Mr. Pott, a very clever neat Surgeon. Home at 9.

54 Rodgers to Rush, London, Aug. 9, 1784. Rush MSS. (L C P, Ridgway), XIV, 132; Hall to Rush, Oct. 18, 1783, in Ruschenberger, *op. cit.*, 16–17.

55 The original journal of Dr. Shippen, covering the period from July 19, 1759, to January 22, 1760, is in the possession of Dr. J. Hall Pleasants, of Baltimore, Md., to whom I wish again to express my grateful appreciation. Dr. Pleasants graciously sent me a typescript copy of the journal to use in the preparation of this paper, and it is from this copy that the quotations are taken. Some entries in the diary were quoted by Dr. J. M. T. Finney in his Hunterian Lecture in London in 1927, "The Influence of John Hunter upon Early American Surgery," *Lancet*, CCXII (Feb. 19, 26, 1927), pt. 1, 420–22, 469–72. The paper was also published as a pamphlet.

The influence of John Hunter on Philip Syng Physick has often been commented upon.[56] With a liberal education in Philadelphia, a three years' apprenticeship to Adam Kuhn, and attendance on the medical lectures at the University of Pennsylvania, Physick went to England in 1789 and was entered by his father as a house pupil with John Hunter. There is a pleasant anecdote, which must be repeated because it reflects the temper of John Hunter and, presumably, that which marked his pupil, to the effect that when the elder Physick inquired what books his son would need, Hunter took him by the arm and leading him to the dissecting room said, "These are the books your son will learn; the others are fit for very little."[57] At once the boy entered upon his work, in May he became a dresser at St. George's Hospital, and in December, probably by the influence of Hunter, was appointed a house surgeon at the Hospital, with an allowance of £25 for board and lodging. As an American, not even a colonial, he encountered the jealousy of the unsuccessful candidates for this post and this put him on his mettle. That jealousy gave way to respect and admiration, however, Randolph tells, when Physick successfully reduced a dislocated shoulder before the entire class of

[56] Unfortunately the journal and letters which Physick wrote during his medical studies abroad cannot be located. They were formerly in the possession of a descendant and were seen by Dr. Francis R. Packard; but upon their owner's death, they could not be found. It is the judgment of Dr. Packard, who inquired carefully after them, that "they are irretrievably lost." Letter to author, Philadelphia, August 26, 1942.

Physick's contemporaries recognized his indebtedness to John Hunter. His son-in-law, Dr. Randolph, spoke of him as "a favorite and attached pupil" of John Hunter and dedicated his *Memoir* of his father-in-law (Phila., 1839) "to the Shade of John Hunter." Though his picture of Jenner and Physick vying as fellow students in Hunter's laboratory is anachronistic, Charles Caldwell, in the *Discourse* on Physick already cited, recognized the importance of the master's teaching. The idea has been repeated and elaborated by George W. Norris, *Early History of Medicine in Philadelphia* (Phila., 1886), 230; William H. Welch, "Influence of English Medicine upon American Medicine in its Formative Period," *Contributions to Medical and Biological Research Dedicated to Sir William Osler* . . . (N. Y., 1919), II, 814; Thomas McCrae in the *Dictionary of American Biography*, XIV, 555; and Sir D'Arcy Power, "How the Tradition of British Surgery Came to America," American Surgical Association, *Transactions*, XLII (1924), 14–27.

[57] Stephen Paget, *John Hunter, Man of Science and Surgeon (1728–1793)* (London, 1897), 233. The elder Physick was asked by Hunter to procure a pair of opossums. After much difficulty Mr. Physick was able to send over a female opossum with her young. He accompanied the gift by a letter containing feeding instructions and the warning that, if the animals must be moved, "they should be lifted by the Tail, or they will bite." Physick to Hunter, Phila., May 20, 1790. Penn-Physick MSS. (H S P), II, 274–75.

medical students.[58] It was during this year of hospital service that Physick performed, at Hunter's request, a series of experiments for the *Treatise on the Blood, Inflammation, and Gun-Shot Wounds* (London, 1794). In this work Hunter recorded his judgment that he could depend on Physick's accuracy.[59] Upon the completion of his year's service at St. George's, Physick returned to Hunter to work, and it was probably at this period that Hunter asked Physick to remain in England and share his practice. Declining what must have been a tempting offer—only Thomas Ruston of all the Philadelphians, it seems, settled in England to practice[60]—Physick went up to Edinburgh, took his degree the next year, attended the practice of the Royal Infirmary there for a few months, and returned to Philadelphia. But to John Hunter he had an indebtedness which he ever acknowledged. Indeed, his son-in-law declared that the admiration Physick had for Hunter "amounted to a species of veneration. Certain it is, that he never ceased to consider him as the greatest man that ever adorned the medical profession."[61]

Such intimate contact as Shippen and Physick had with John Hunter, and which other students enjoyed in greater or less degree with other physicians and surgeons, was one of the best ways to acquire medical knowledge and the cream of medical experience. Perhaps it was the memory of the benefits received from his attendance at the weekly sessions Sir John Pringle held at his home for a select group of medical students, that made Rush advise his pupils in turn to "gain access to & cultivate an intimacy wth a few eminent physicians & surgeons—you will profit more by asking them questions in a few hours, than by attending hospital practice for years."[62] That this professor-student relation might be pleasant and profitable is attested by the picture which Professor Fabricius, of Kiel, Kuhn's fellow student at Upsala, drew of their almost idyllic life together

58 Randolph, *op. cit.*, 24–25; George Edwards, "Philip Syng Physick, 1768–1837," Royal Medical Society, *Proceedings*, XXXIII (1939–40), pt. 1, 145–46.

59 The note is on page 95*n*. It is quoted in Middleton, "Philip Syng Physick: Father of American Surgery," *Annals of Medical History*, n.s., I (1929), 564.

60 Samuel Bard to John Morgan, New York, Nov. 16, 1767. Carson, *op. cit.*, II, 13. The copy of a journal which Dr. Ruston kept in France in 1785 is in The Historical Society of Pennsylvania.

61 Randolph, *op. cit.*, 28, 30–31.

62 Rush, "Letters, Facts & Observations upon a Variety of Subjects," 47–51. Rush MSS. (L C P, Ridgway).

with Linnaeus. Not a day passed that they did not see him, either at lectures or in familiar conversations. "In summer we followed him into the country. We were three, Kuhn, Zoega, and I, all foreigners. In winter we lived directly facing his house, and he came to us almost every day, in his short red *robe de chambre*, with a green fur-cap on his head and a pipe in his hand. He came for half an hour but stopped a whole one, and many times two."[63] And Linnaeus, when Kuhn was about to leave Europe, wrote to him in terms seldom used by a teacher of a student, saying that he cherished him "as a beloved son, for your correct and engaging deportment, in which none of the foreigners excelled you; for your unwearied ardor and application in cultivating the sciences, in which you were surpassed by no one; for your undisguised friendship, in which none could have equalled you."[64] Similarly Cullen had a high opinion of his American students: he constantly cited Morgan's diligence and reputation as an encouragement of the other American students,[65] and resuming his correspondence after the American War he told Rush, "I hold you and shall always hold you in the same esteem and affection as ever." Then he sent his "respectful and affectionate compliments to all my old pupils at Philadelphia. I shall always hold it my highest honour that the founders of the Medical College of Philadelphia were all of them my Pupils and if it can be known I think it will be the most certain means of transmitting my name to a distant posterity for I believe that this School will one day or other be the greatest in the world."[66]

Naturally the students compared the opportunities for study in Europe with those they had known at the Edinburgh of America; and they concluded that on the whole the formal instruction at Philadelphia was not inferior to that found anywhere in Europe. Only when he visited the Hunters' anatomical museum was Thomas Parke ashamed for his native city, and he "blushed for ye indolence & neglect of our Philad^a Professor of Anatomy—for sure a more com-

---

63 D. H. Stoever, *The Life of Sir Charles Linnaeus* . . . (London, 1794), 273–74. This is quoted in part by Willis L. Jepson in his sketch of Kuhn in the *Dictionary of American Biography*, X, 511.

64 Linnaeus to Kuhn, Upsala, Feb. 20, 1767. "Biographical Notice of Dr. Adam Kuhn," *Eclectic Repertory* . . ., VIII (1818), 247.

65 Rush to Morgan, Edinburgh, Nov. 16, 1766. Gratz Collection (H S P), Case 1, Box 20.

66 Cullen to Rush, Edinburgh, Oct. 16, 1784. Rush MSS. (L C P, Ridgway), XXIV, 56.

plete collection of preparations I think is not in Europe. Nay every
part of the Human Body is there to be Seen in its greatest beauty
—instead of an old dirty Theatre I there beheld the most elegant
building suitable for the purpose—in short it so far surpasses anything of the kind I ever saw before y^t. I think I cannot wth. any
patience ever enter Shippens hereafter."[67] Particulars aside, however, the general judgment was favorable to the American work.
Griffitts often told Rodgers that he received more satisfaction and
improvement from his medical masters in Philadelphia than in
France or England.[68] Rodgers was "somewhat disappointed in my
high raised expectations of its [England's] Medical Perfections—I am
persuaded that Medicine is taught more Scientifically in Philad^a. than
in London, & that our Teachers there are more attentive to the
improvement of their Pupils than they are here."[69] Barton was, as
he wrote from Edinburgh, "convinced, by experience, that little is
wanted in Philadelphia to make that school one of the first seats of
medicine in the world."[70] In Germany Foulke found that "the coolness with which Science is courted at Leipsic & a general disposition
to a contentment in such discoveries as the Sons of Science in France
or Great Britain may throw into the world, tends to continue old
usages, & Theories, & such parts of the School of Leipsic, as I have
at present acquaintance with appear much inferior to that of Paris
& no way superior to that young Seminary" which owed its birth to
his correspondent Dr. Franklin.[71] As if to place a kind of seal upon
these opinions, Daniel Coxe, who was, however, more American than
English, sent his son John Redman Coxe to study medicine with
Dr. Rush at Philadelphia, where, he thought, the "lights & practical
aids" of physic could be better got than in England, to which the
boy would return for the final touches.[72]

The impression of hard work which the letters and journals of
these Philadelphia students of medicine give is probably well founded.
Yet, after the manner of medical students of every age, they had
their ways of recreation and diversion; and few could have failed to

67 Parke, Journal, No. 1, July 31, 1771. Pemberton Papers (H S P), LVII, 93.
68 Rodgers to Rush, London, July 7, 1784. Rush MSS. (L C P, Ridgway), XIV, 133.
69 Rodgers to Rush, London, Aug. 9, 1784. Rush MSS. (L C P, Ridgway), XIV, 132.
70 Barton to Rush, Edinburgh, Jan. 24, 1787. Rush MSS. (L C P, Ridgway), XXVII, 2.
71 Foulke to Franklin, Leipsic, Oct. 12, 1781. Franklin Papers (APS), XXIII, 11.
72 Coxe to Rush, London, May 16, 1791. Rush MSS. (L C P, Ridgway), XXVII, 11.

appreciate Rush's cry as he left Edinburgh, that "the happiest period of my Life is now near over, my Halcyon Days have been spent in Edin."[73] George Logan, when he was sent by Dr. Fothergill to Dunmow, forty miles from London, to work for a year with a country practitioner, found the place "a properer situation for an Anchoret, than a human being who has the least taste for a social life."[74] But Edinburgh and London especially were more lively. At very least there were the usual sights to see. Within a few weeks of his arrival in the English metropolis Parke visited St. James' and Buckingham palaces, saw the menagerie at the Tower and the elephants at Buckingham House—"ye largest & most frightfull Beasts I ever saw." He walked through the elegant and enchanting gardens of Vaux Hall, and was charmed by the lawns and paths and pools of Kensington Gardens. He learned that two hours were not enough to examine the British Museum's "most amasing collection of Curiosities"; he climbed up to the tower of St. Paul's to get a view of London; and he climbed out of bed one morning at half past five to go to Blackheath to see the King, the Duke of Gloucester, and the Prince of Wales at a military review, "a most grand sight," thought this Philadelphia Quaker. And there were brief excursions to make. Guide book in hand, Parke went to Oxford, where he found "one of the most curious Cities in England"; he visited Bath, as did George Logan, and, like Logan, he used only superlatives to describe it. Plays and lectures found the Philadelphians in attendance. Shippen saw Garrick several times, in Macbeth, which he thought "surprising"; in Lear, which he thought "inimitable"; and from France he carried back to Garrick a personal letter from Laurence Sterne.[75] He heard Whitefield preach on a number of occasions, as did Rush at least once. Franklin took him to the Royal Society. On another occasion at the College of Physicians he heard Mark Akenside, physician and poet, read a "very entertaining" paper on Harvey. There were the pleasures of the table and, sometimes, of the bottle too; for no American went to England and the Continent without letters to friends and relatives who delighted to entertain them and

---

[73] Rush to Morgan, Edinburgh, July 27, 1768. Carson, op. cit., II, 27.

[74] Logan to Charles Logan, Dunmow, Aug. 16, 1775. Letter Book (H S P).

[75] Lewis Perry Curtis, editor, Letters of Laurence Sterne (Oxford, 1935), 156. This reference was suggested by Herbert Thoms, "William Shippen, Jr., the Great Pioneer in American Obstetrics," American Journal of Obstetrics and Gynecology, XXXVII (1939), 514.

whom, sometimes, it profited them to be with. Rush called once on John Wilkes, whose library of "histories and commonplace literature" he thought mirrored the trivial character of the man. With his fellow-Pennsylvanian Benjamin West he spent several pleasant evenings and met Sir Joshua Reynolds; and Reynolds invited him to dine one day with Oliver Goldsmith and the massive Dr. Johnson.[76] One night at Sir John Shaw's seat, Shippen was one of a party that sat drinking claret until midnight and then "retired and bedded, much pleased"; and it was Shippen who, more than twenty years after he left Edinburgh, when he was sending back one of his own students, recalled himself to Cullen as "a pupil who was as fond of a Solan Goose as you were."[77]

Finally, of course, there were the ladies. Shippen frequently interrupted his anatomical studies with the Hunters to attend a dance. Some of these occasions were made pleasant for him by his fair companions. Others he set down—like an honest Philadelphian—as being conducted without order or regularity. For Dr. Parke the date December 14, 1771, must have been a sort of red-letter day, for he then "saw some very fine Women for ye first [time] in Edinburgh that I tho't any thing like Venus's." Perhaps Betsy Empson was such a Venus; at any rate, after spending an evening with her, Parke wrote remorsefully into his journal, "Cou'd medical knowledge be acquired in this manner I think I should soon be a proficient, but alas! I fear I am wrong in not being more diligent." What John Foulke learned about women, older women at least, is only hinted at by the query of his friend George Fox, whether Foulke was "as assiduous as heretofore in his visits to the *bald Head and Tail Countess* [possibly Mme. la Comtesse de la Mark], or has he forfeited by some inconstancy the honorable title of *mon Fils*."[78] And apparently in London one could always, if one wished, as Thomas Parke did not, be "captivated by ye Ladies which so plentifully are planted all along the Strand to entice young Gentlemen home w^th.

76 Goodman, *op. cit.*, 18–19.

77 Shippen to Cullen, Phila., April 27, 1784, in John D. Comrie, "An Eighteenth Century Consultant," *Medical Life*, XXXII (1925), 137.

78 Fox to William Temple Franklin, St. Florentin, July 10, 1781. Franklin Papers (A P S), CIII, 72.

them." All in all, it was probably not a life of unrelieved application to studies.[79]

Something of what European study meant to the professional training of the young doctors from Philadelphia, European travel meant to the broadening of their general experience. New places, new faces, and new ideas all opened up a different world from that which revolved in ordered paths around the city on the Delaware. Not content to see of Europe only what they viewed from the windows of their lecture halls and laboratories, they set out to make a grand tour of the Continent. When his work at Edinburgh, London, and Paris was finished, procuring a copy of Thomas Nugent's *The Grand Tour*, Morgan made a trip to Italy, visiting the art galleries and noting the names of the works displayed, entering the churches and casting a skeptical eye on the miracles allegedly performed in some of them, and meeting a few of the great and near-great and some of more interesting residents of that ancient land.[80] Shippen, despite the war, was able to get to France in the capacity of physician to Louisa Poyntz, sister of Lady Spencer.[81] Kuhn, who studied in Sweden, Scotland, and England, traveled also in France, Holland, and Germany. Not only did they receive new impressions and make the acquaintance of persons different from those they knew at home in Philadelphia, but the European experience wore away some of the angularities of their manners. John Foulke, for example, during the period of his service as a Revolutionary Army surgeon, was described by a fellow surgeon as "a pedantic young Quaker"; but, if the letters of his gay friends William Temple Franklin and George Fox mirror

[79] The matter of these paragraphs comes primarily from the Journal of Thomas Parke, Pemberton Papers (H S P), LVII, 93–98, and from the Journal of William Shippen, Junior, in the possession of Dr. Pleasants.

[80] Morgan's was the most ambitious of the tours, and his reputation and acquaintance paved the way for others who came after him. Griffitts, for example, stayed with the very family in Paris with whom Morgan had lived twenty years before. But Morgan himself followed partly in the wake of two fellow-Philadelphians. From Naples on May 12, 1764, he wrote to Joseph Shippen, Junior, that "amongst ten thousand english Men whose Names are inscribed on ye Walls of Nero's Prison," he and Samuel Powel, his traveling companion, "descry'd Yours & M^r. Allen's in legible Characters." (Balch Collection, Shippen Papers (H S P), I, 127.) One wonders whether, in the manner of tourists of that and later days, Dr. John Morgan, M.D. and soon to be F.R.S., left his autograph for other Philadelphians to find.

The original of Morgan's journal of his Continental trip is in the University of Pennsylvania Medical School.

[81] Curtis, editor, *Letters of Laurence Sterne*, 156.

him accurately, in Europe he deserved anything but the epithet "pedantic." To be sure, simply traveling a bit into Europe, even meeting some of the great and dining at their tables, as Morgan did with the Duke of York in Italy, was no earnest of broadened intellectual horizons or high resolves taken. But the experience had this worth, that it gave the young colonists and the new republicans a certain self-confidence which stood them and their profession in good stead, it introduced them to their fellow workers in medicine, and it gave them a pipe line into that bubbling cauldron of ideas which marked Europe at the century's close.

In the journals they kept and in the letters they wrote home they recorded their impressions of England and of Europe and they made their judgments, profound or ill-considered, of the places and the people they saw. Of course there was the weather. From Phineas Bond, a law student with whom some of the medical students often dined, English weather received its due: "There is such a continued Fog in this Country, that the Sun does not appear once a Month," he grumbled. "They call it fine Weather if it is possible to walk half a Mile without being wet to ye Skin."[82] Britain's weather was indeed discouraging, for hardly an American came to that land to study who did not fall ill. Caspar Wistar felt his sickness had so far retarded his advancement that he half considered returning home without his degree:[83] and it was to the illness and convalescence of Benjamin Smith Barton that his friends owed his *Observations on Natural History*. The weather of Paris was equally condemned by Griffitts, who gave it as one of the reasons for studying at Montpellier that in southern France the sun shone for days on end, "which to a Person coming from the Bogs of Paris forms a very agreeable Contrast."[84]

For the cities, especially the English cities, their enthusiasm was equally restrained. Probably it was the uniqueness of Venice, rather than its beauty, that made Morgan speak of it as "rising out of the Sea . . . indeed a beautiful object";[85] and though Logan spoke of London as "this grand superb City," he noted in Dover the narrow

---

82 Bond to Samuel Rhoads, London, Dec. 28, 1771. (MS., College of Physicians of Phila.).

83 Wistar to Thomas Wistar, Edinburgh, Feb. 14, 1785. Vaux Papers (H S P).

84 Griffitts to M. and H. Griffitts, Montpellier, Jan. 7, 1783. Griffitts Correspondence (H S P); Griffitts to William Temple Franklin, Montpellier, Oct. 31, 1782. Franklin Papers (A P S), CIV, 118.

85 Morgan, *Journal*, 113.

and irregular streets and the houses "by no means elegant," thought
Colchester "badly built and worse paved," and, like other medical
students in that northern capital, was impressed by "the remarkable
filthiness" of Edinburgh.[86] It was a "nasty Town," thought Dr. John
Sims, Logan's preceptor and Parke's friend,[87] where, as Benjamin
Rush observed, not without some humor, there was an intimate
connection between sanitation and the franchise. The houses of
Edinburgh having neither yards nor cellars and so no necessary
houses, "all their filth of every kind is thrown out of their windows.
This is done in the night generally, and is carried away next morning
by carts appointed for that purpose. Unhappy they who are obliged
to walk out after ten or eleven o'clock at night. It is no uncommon
thing to receive what Juvenal says he did, in his first satire, from a
window in Rome. This is called here being *naturalized*. As yet I have
happily escaped being made a freeman of the city in this way, but
my unfortunate friend Potts has gained the honour before me."[88]
L'Orient, Griffitts' first sight of France and a French town, presented
an agreeable variety "to a Person who has seen nothing above the
plain & elegant Streets of Philadelphia. . . . The Houses to be sure
are old fashioned & all of Stone but if they do not look elegant they
look venerable, & we have plenty of Gothic Churches Castles &c."[89]
But there was no nonsense about Griffitts. To a young friend in
Philadelphia who seems to have been sighing for a glimpse of the
Old World, he wrote like a philosopher, "Let me tell you for your
Comfort that the little Alley you live in, is far preferable in some
respects to many of the largest Streets in Paris—To be sure the
Houses are not 6 or 7 Stories high but then a Person can walk
without getting up to their Knees in Mud—"[90] London he dismissed
summarily: "The Palaces are nothing at all, as to the outside—The
Park is so, so—Perhaps a dozen good looking houses, and so much
for London."[91]

[86] Logan to Charles Logan, London, July 9, 1775; Dunmow, June 29, 1776; Edinburgh,
Feb. 2, 1777. Letter Book (H S P).

[87] Sims to Parke, Edinburgh, May 13, 1772. Pemberton Papers, Parrish Collection (H S P).

[88] Rush to [——], [Edinburgh], Dec. 29, 1766. *Notes and Queries*, X (1854), 520.

[89] Griffitts to Abigail Griffitts, L'Orient, Sept. 9, 1781. Griffitts Correspondence (H S P).

[90] Griffitts to [——], Paris, Oct. 1, 1781. MS. Collection of Library Company of Philadelphia.

[91] Griffitts to Mrs. O'Connor, London, Aug. 10, 1783. Carson, *op. cit.*, II, 107.

Their reaction to the countryside was quite different. As he traveled northward from London to Edinburgh, Logan made careful note of the agricultural improvements generally in evidence. With the eye of an agricultural reformer he described the rural districts he passed through and his comments and descriptions reveal the interest and intelligence that were to make the Stenton farm a model. Everywhere he found agriculture "carried on with great spirit, and with such advantage that many in this Neighbourhood [Dunmow] have made large fortunes"; and he cited the instance of a gentleman who was said to have amassed £20,000 in thirty years by his attention to farming alone. In Scotland he found the same spirit prevailing. There Lord Kames was intensely interested in agriculture which had "nearly become a polite part of education, and is generally the topic of conversation among those of the first characters."[92]

But one did not need to be an agriculturist to be charmed by the beauties of the English or European scene, and many of the Philadelphians revealed in their letters a deep appreciation of them. Shippen, for example, wrote in his journal of walking out to the seat of Lord Tinley at Wanstead, which had "before it a grand lawn beset with Marble Images and Lamps, at the End of it a piece of water 11 Acres. On one side a fine woody Grove with a great Stream of Water running thro it etc. very pretty."[93] But this was artificial. What Morgan saw in Italy was real and the romantic appreciation of this man of science flashes through the awkwardness of his grammar and the inadequacy of his vocabulary. The cascade of Terni was "a most astonishing and sublime sight," its waters tumbling "in a white foamy Column; ye circling ringlets following each other in quick succession like lightning glance on ye eye of the spectator." The Alps, he thought, seemed "to overtop the very Clouds, shewing their hoary heads in the clear Azure expanse of the Firmament many & many leagues, towering aloft, & stretching along the Horrizon in a Chain as far as the Eye could reach. . . ." From Mount Cenis "a rude but sublime Picture presented itself all round—Hills highing their Heads in Clouds—Some seeming to pierce, & seem above the Clouds in the upper regions of Air covered with snow—Water pre-

92 Logan to Charles Logan, Dunmow, Aug. 16, 1775; Bristol, Sept. 22, 1776; Edinburgh, Dec. 16, 1776, July, 1778. Letter Book (H S P).

93 Shippen, Journal, Sept. 3, 1759. (Typescript copy in possession of Dr. Pleasants.)

cipitating itself down the sides of the Hills forming innumerable Cascades & running with impetuous force to the foot of the Hill."[94]

Naturally the travelers passed the people of Europe in judgment before them. Logan liked the Scots: the Highlanders, though inquisitive and superstitious, were hospitable, brave, generous, and sensitive of their honor; the lower classes he thought honest and generally sober, though dirty in their houses and persons; while the education and easy bearing of the Scottish ladies made them, he thought, "fit companions for Men of sense."[95] Parke's chief complaint against the people of North Britain was that they prepared their food "in ye Scotch Taste, i.e. one third Dirt by way of Condiment."[96] On the whole, however, though Morgan had some things to say on the morality of Italian women and Rush made an honest but not entirely successful effort to divest himself of inherited prejudices against those of France, the Philadelphians were remarkably slow to make a comprehensive judgment of any national character. It was the part of a philosopher to try to comprehend.

The American Revolution seems to have influenced the reception the English gave the Americans and also the Americans' attitude toward the English. It appears certain that the medical students who went abroad before 1775 met on the whole with a friendlier treatment, entered more freely into the social life of that country, and made acquaintances and friends more easily than did those who went to England after 1783. For to these, since they were no longer colonials, the English felt less responsibility and they betrayed a certain restraint and formality which irked the Americans. Griffitts put it succinctly: "They are not extravagantly fond of Americans in England, tho' they generally behave very politely when conversing on Politicks." Others carried away the same impression.[97] Of course, war or no war, those with relations or other intimate ties in England continued to find a welcome. The position of the elder Physick and his services to the Penn family opened many doors to his son; Logan

94 Morgan, *Journal*, 62, 171, 207.
95 Logan to Charles Logan, Edinburgh, June 1, 1777, Feb. 27, 1778. Letter Book (H S P).
96 Parke, Journal, No. 2, Oct. 26, 1771. Pemberton Papers (H S P), LVII, 98.
97 Griffitts to Mrs. O'Connor, London, Aug. 10, 1783. Carson, *op. cit.*, II, 107; James Hall to Rush, Hastings, Sept. 7, 1783. Rush MSS. (L C P, Ridgway), XXXIII, 104.

bore an impressive name among Friends;[98] while the English seem
never to have ignored ability and social grace.

Occasionally these young travelers from the Quaker City touched
the skirts of fame and greatness. Rush saw the royal family dine
publicly at Versailles but was shocked to see the Dauphin take a
piece of meat from his mouth, look at it carefully, and throw it on
the floor.[99] In London Morgan and Shippen, "with a couple of
Ladies," saw the coronation procession of George III. Morgan cast
an appraising eye over the figure of the Queen—"rather a little
woman than otherwise," not beautiful but sweet and affable in appearance, "a fine slender waist, her carriage, air & manners incom-
parably easy, & genteel; I think majestic—upon ye whole an amiable
woman to look at . . . ."[100] In Rome Morgan had another treat.
Arriving there in the party of the Duke of York, he was invited to
all the entertainments given for His Royal Highness, even dined at
his table on a sturgeon sent the Duke with the papal blessing. He
had a private audience with His Holiness—"he was affable and
courteous," the erstwhile Quaker reported—and during Holy Week
attended one of "ye grand functions at wch the Pope assists in Person
—next to ye Coronation tis one of the finest sights I ever saw."[101]
But the choicest treat was yet in store. On his way back to Paris
and to Philadelphia Morgan and his fellow traveler, Samuel Powel,
paid a visit to the Sage of Ferney. They spent several hours with
Voltaire and when in the evening they took their leave, they received
a thunderous farewell: "Behold two Amiable Young Men," the great
man declaimed before his company, pointing to the Philadelphians,
"Lovers of Truth & Inquirers into Nature. They are not satisfy'd
with mear Appearances, they love Investigation & Truth, & despize
Superstition—I commend You Gentlemen—go on, love Truth &

98 Edmund Physick to Mrs. Richard Penn, Phila., Jan. 1, 1790. Penn-Physick MSS.
(H S P), II, 256; Logan to Charles Logan, Edinburgh, Nov. 17, 1776. Letter Book (H S P);
[——] Bush to Parke, London, March 3, 1789. Gilbert Collection of MS. Letters (College of
Physicians of Phila.), I, 289.

99 Goodman, op. cit., 22.

100 Morgan to Joseph Shippen, Junior, London, Oct. 12, 1761. Shippen Papers (H S P), V,
167.

101 Morgan to Joseph Shippen, Junior, Naples, May 12, 1764. Balch Collection, Shippen
Papers (H S P), I, 127; Morgan, Journal, 26.

search diligently after it. Hate Hypocrisy Hate Masses & above all hate the Priests."[102]

And so finally, their studies completed, their travels at an end, they returned home, these Philadelphians, to practice and to teach. For, whether it was something that Europe gave them or something that Europe had only prepared them to do, teach they must and teach they did. A surprising number were imbued with a passion to bring medical knowledge to America; like Griffitts they returned home "with an high Idea of our University."[103] Morgan, Shippen, Rush, and Kuhn formed the first faculty of the medical school; and Wistar, Griffitts, Barton, and Physick joined it subsequently. John H. Gibbons gave private lectures on theory and practice after 1789.[104] Foulke, becoming interested in balloons, delivered popular lectures on pneumatics and offered courses in anatomy, so that one of his friends jestingly called him both the Montgolfier and the Monro of America;[105] and Rodgers, leaving Philadelphia after a few years, went to New York, where he taught in the medical school of that city. Of almost every one of these Philadelphia students of medicine one might say that he proved to be, as Dr. Franklin predicted of Morgan, "of great Use to his Country as well as an Honour to the Medical School of Edinburgh."[106]

[102] Morgan, *Journal*, 216–29.

[103] John R. B. Rodgers to Rush, London, July 7, 1784. Rush MSS. (L C P, Ridgway), XIV, 133.

[104] G. W. Norris, *op. cit.*, 122.

[105] John Sims to Parke, London, June 15, 1784. Gilbert Collection of MS. Letters (College of Physicians of Phila.), IV, 81; H. M. Lippincott, "Dr. John Foulke, 1780, a Pioneer in Aeronautics," *General Magazine and Historical Chronicle*, XXXIV (1932), 528.

[106] Franklin to Sir Alexander Dick, London, June 2, 1765, in Pepper, "The Medical Side of Benjamin Franklin," *loc. cit.*, 214–15.

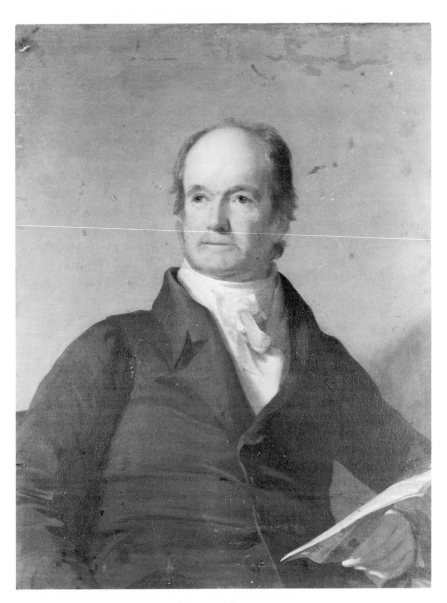

Thomas Parke

Thomas Parke, M.B., Physician and Friend

THOMAS PARKE was not a great man. A practicing physician for more than sixty years and a member of the staff of the Pennsylvania Hospital for more than forty, he made no medical discovery or invention, devised no policy that was clearly his, and left a reputation for cautious practice and solid worth that was a greater tribute to his character than to his learning. As president of the College of Physicians of Philadelphia he is remembered chiefly because his reign was one of the longest in its history. When he died the College heard a eulogy spoken, as it was in duty bound to do; since that day more than a century ago almost nothing has been said of him except by genealogically-inclined descendants less interested in him, be it said, than in the families he was connected with by marriage.

If Parke was not a great man, neither was he an indispensable one. The several institutions he served so faithfully and long—the Hospital, the Library Company, and the College of Physicians—as the years of his connection with them passed thirty, then forty, must sometimes have thought him coeval with themselves. But when at last ill health forced him to retire from some posts and death removed him from others, his going was scarcely felt. There were the usual expressions of regret and the usual testimonies to faithful service; and that was all. The truth is there were dozens of persons in Philadelphia quite as able as Thomas Parke to do what he did as a physician and a citizen.

Neither great nor indispensable, he was thus a man of the second rank. The world is filled with such people. Yet these men's lives have meaning. The Franklins and the Jeffersons on the one hand, the scoundrels and the killers on the other, are all well known; they crowd history's galleries. But it is the large body of unimaginative, undistinguished men of the middle sort who do most of the world's work. It is they who keep alive the ideas other men conceive and hold together the institutions other men create. They serve laboriously on committees, collect money for good causes, and preach and teach and write for the largest audience. They originate little; they transmit much. They are the ideal trustees, the perfect friends. They are the useful ones, like Thomas Parke.

He came of an honest, hard-working, prosperous Quaker stock. His grandfather Thomas, a farmer in Ireland where he owned his own land, quitted his homeland when he was sixty years of age and came to America in 1724 with his wife and seven of his ten children. The family stayed a few months in Chester in Penn's province, then purchased a tract of five hundred acres in the Great Valley in East Caln Township, Chester County, where a modest but sturdy stone house was built. It is still standing on a slight eminence near the Lancaster Pike, facing eastward toward the Quaker capital at Philadelphia, overlooking the gently rolling Chester countryside. The seventh son of this Irish Quaker immigrant, named Thomas for his father, was nineteen when the family came to Pennsylvania. For several years he helped his father on the farm. Subsequently he was proprietor of the Ship Tavern on the road near the family homestead; of him it was written that "although he kept a public house, he was adorned with so much regularity, that he gave content to most civilized persons, that called at his house." [1] A respected citizen and landowner, he was one of the inhabitants of the townships of Caln, Whiteland, and Uwchlan who signed petitions to the provincial governor in 1736 and 1737 asking for a review of the survey recently made of a road leading from Paxtang on the Susquehanna to Philadelphia. [2] This Thomas Parke had seven children, three sons, three daughters, and a girl who died in infancy. The fifth child and second son was Thomas, third of that name in America, the subject of this sketch. [3]

He was born in East Caln Township on August 6, 1749. By birthright a member of Bradford Monthly Meeting, his Friendly inheritance and upbringing were distinguishing elements in his character and career. "He

[1] James P. Parke, "An Account of the Parke Family," typescript copy in the possession of Ellis Y. Brown, Jr., of Downingtown, Pa. Mr. Brown lives in the house of Thomas Parke the immigrant.

[2] Provincial Papers, VI, 43, VII, 28, Archives Division, Pennsylvania Historical and Museum Commission, Harrisburg.

[3] Henry D. Biddle, *A Sketch of Owen Biddle, to which is added a short account of the Parke family* ... (Privately printed, Phila., 1892), 39-46.

was blessed," declared his eulogist before the College of Physicians more than eighty years later, "with an excellent constitution, which the active and simple habits of his early country life tended to confirm." [4] In certain ways, indeed, Parke was always a plain country Friend. Before he was ten his father died, but the family was not left in straitened circumstances. As for young Thomas, his father's will suggests a special regard for him: he received his father's plantation—the eldest son Robert took an adjoining farm; he received his father's oldest desk—Robert took the newest; and, when he became twenty-one, Thomas was to get his father's watch.[5] Two years after his father's death, while he was living with his widowed mother, his oldest sister Sarah married. Her husband was Owen Biddle, clock- and watch-maker of Philadelphia, an enthusiast for science, later one of the founders of the American Philosophical Society. To "O.B.," as after the Friendly fashion he so generally appears in Thomas' letters and journal, Thomas Parke became deeply attached; he loved and respected him, sought and followed his advice. It was probably Biddle who, discerning young Thomas' promise and in furtherance of the family's purpose, brought the boy to Philadelphia, provided for him while he studied there, and encouraged him toward medicine. In any case, leaving his local Chester County school, Thomas came to Philadelphia to enter the classical school of Robert Proud and begin the study of medicine under Dr. Cadwalader Evans. On December 12, 1766, Parke received a certificate from the Bradford Monthly Meeting to the Philadelphia Monthly Meeting.[6] He was a Philadelphian from this time forward.

Parke's medical preceptor was one of the constant stars in that bright galaxy of medical practitioners and teachers who gave Philadelphia so much of its reputation in the international world of science in the latter half of the eighteenth century. Evans had begun his medical studies with Dr. Thomas Bond in Philadelphia; he had continued them at London. With his friend Benjamin Franklin as technician, he once employed

[4] Joseph Parrish, "Biographical Notice of Dr Thomas Parke read before the College of Physicians, June 7, 1836," in Biographical sketches and memoirs of members of the College of Physicians of Philadelphia, 5-8, MS, College of Physicians of Philadelphia.

[5] Thomas Parke, Will, 10 mo. 15, 1758, contemporary copy, Pemberton Papers, XII, 159, Historical Society of Pennsylvania. The Historical Society will be referred to hereafter as HSP.

[6] William Wade Hinshaw, Encyclopedia of American Quaker Genealogy (Ann Arbor, Mich., 1938), II, 613.

electricity in a case of convulsions which he reported to the *London
Medical Journal*. He was one of Franklin's correspondents and one of the
founders of the American Philosophical Society. Since 1759 he had been
a physician at the Pennsylvania Hospital.

Most of Parke's time was spent reading and working under his master's
direction, but Dr. Evans did direct his pupil to enroll for medical lectures
in the College of Philadelphia. Accordingly Parke took one course of
lectures the first year, 1767. It was anatomy under Dr. William Shippen,
Jr.; he paid the instructor six pistoles. In the spring he attended the botany
lectures of Dr. Adam Kuhn, newly-returned from Edinburgh and from
study with Linnaeus at Upsala. The next season Parke repeated Shippen's
course in anatomy, took Kuhn's course on materia medica and pharmacy,
and attended the work in chemistry and the theory and practice of physic-
of "John Morgan MD, FRS and Profr. of the Theory and Practice of
Medicine," as that gentleman signed himself on the back of the playing
card which served as ticket of admission to the course. The third year,
1769, Parke kept up his work in chemistry, now under Dr. Benjamin
Rush. He continued in theory and practice, where his card of admission
now described him as a "perpetual pupil," and he went ahead in practical
midwifery with Thomas Bond at the Hospital.[7] Parke's notes which have
survived indicate that he was an intelligent student. In a little compilation
of chemical facts, for example, though he extracted materials from Mac-
quer's *Elements of the Theory and Practice of Chemistry* (second edition,
1764), he rearranged them to suit his purpose as a student. To prepare for
his final examination he attended the public examinations of the medical
candidates the year before he was to receive his degree and carefully
noted all the questions asked.[8] Completing his work after three years, he
was graduated on June 5, 1770, with the degree of bachelor of medicine,
the only medical graduate that year. Provost Smith delivered "a very
interesting Charge to the Graduates"; and the Reverend Mr. George
Whitefield, who was present, "concluded the whole, at the Request of the
Faculty, with an excellent and catholic Prayer," which doubtless embraced

---

[7] Parke's tickets of admission are in the library of the School of Medicine of the
University of Pennsylvania. Thomas Bond, "List of Clinical Pupils, April 11, 1770,"
MS. Collection, Pennsylvania Hospital.

[8] [Thomas Parke], "Of the Principles of Bodies," MS., College of Physicians of
Philadelphia.

the lone medical graduate, to whom the customary special charge was not delivered.[9]

Though his formal work at the College had thus successfully ended, Parke remained in the city during the fall and winter. He took Rush's course in chemistry a second time and he enrolled for Bond's clinical lectures at the Hospital. To this period belongs an essay on a case of pleuripneumonia in the Alms House; he prepared it, presumably, for the students' medical society.[10] But only in Edinburgh and London was a perfection of medical knowledge to be obtained. Parke decided to go abroad. When he sailed in May 1771 he had provided that his certificate to the Grace Church Street Meeting should be sent him, to open the doors of the Quaker society to him; and he bore a pouchful of letters from his Philadelphia friends and teachers to friends and teachers in London and Edinburgh. Dr. Morgan, who sat up until dawn writing letters of recommendation and other notes to his English friends, introduced Parke to Dr. William Hewson as one who "is modest, ingenuous, diligent in Study, and burns with desire to distinguish himself in his Profession." Shippen recommended him to Hewson as "sensible and clever." Parke's friend William Smith, the new English apothecary at the Hospital, informed a friend that Parke went abroad "to improve himself not only in Medicine, but with Men, Manners and Things." Dr. Morgan's final advice to the young man was to return to Philadelphia to get his doctorate, but in this as in all other matters to follow the advice of Dr. John Fothergill, friend and counselor of American medical students in London in the third quarter of the century.[11]

After a voyage of five weeks during which he was sick almost constantly, Parke reached Bristol on July 5.[12] Here he spent ten days pleasantly with friends and relatives, viewing the town and making some excursions into the neighboring countryside. With a small party he visited Bath, where he stared at "one of the first places in England for Regularity and

[9] *Pennsylvania Gazette*, June 14, 1770.

[10] [Thomas Parke], "[Lecture on a case of pleuripneumonia]," Phila., Nov. 17, 1770, MS., College of Physicians of Philadelphia.

[11] Hinshaw, *Encyclopedia*, II, 613; Shippen to Hewson, Phila., May 24, 1771, in Joseph Carson, *History of the Medical Department of the College of Philadelphia* (Phila., 1869), I, 127; MS. Scrapbook, College of Physicians of Philadelphia; Morgan to Fothergill, Phila., May 24, 1771; William Smith to William Curtis, [Phila.], May 24, 1771, Copies of recommendations of Thomas Parke, Pemberton Papers, Parrish Collection, HSP.

[12] Thomas Parke, "Journal," Pemberton Papers, LVII, 93-98.

high Life," concluding that though the city was worth a visit it was not a place he should care to live in. Everywhere he met members of the tight-knit Quaker society who received him and passed him on to their friends and relatives in other places. From Bristol he proceeded by stage to London, where he found lodging with James Freeman, a Friend. At once Parke presented his letters of introduction to Fothergill. Fothergill advised him to walk the hospital wards, and accordingly took the young man to St. Thomas' Hospital where he introduced him to the physicians, especially Dr. Huck. A few days later, paying 21 guineas for the privilege, he registered as a physician-pupil under Huck at St. Thomas'. At the same time he enrolled in a course in obstetrics taught by Dr. McKenzie, who had been Shippen's teacher.

Parke remained in London until the middle of the fall. During these three months the young man was occupied by his medical studies—McKenzie's lectures began at seven each morning and Parke was due at St. Thomas' at eleven—and by the pleasant associations of the Quaker circle into which he was introduced. Keeping his wits about him, he made interesting comparisons with medical instruction at Philadelphia. At Dr. Hunter's anatomical museum he "blushed for the indolence and neglect of our Philadelphia Professor of Anatomy—for sure a more complete collection of preparations I think is not in Europe. Nay every part of the Human Body is there to be seen in its greatest beauty—instead of an old dirty Theater I there beheld the most Elegant building suitable for the purpose—in short it so far surpasses anything of the kind I ever saw before that I think I cannot with any patience ever enter Shippens hereafter." The dressers whom he watched at St. Thomas' he thought surpassed those of the Pennsylvania Hospital "neither in neatness nor simplicity." He went regularly to Friends meeting, especially to Grace Church Street Meeting, to which his certificate from Philadelphia was addressed, and he came in time to call it his own. Nor did he neglect to see the sights of the city. Generally he described them in superlatives. Hardly had he reached London before he climbed to the top of St. Paul's from which he had "an extensive prospect of the City." He went several times to the British Museum, where the collection of curiosities was the "most amasing" he ever beheld. Although some of the palaces were architecturally disappointing to him, their paintings were "the best I think I ever saw." And he also saw other sights of London, like "the Ladies which so plentifully are planted all along the Strand to entice young Gentlemen home with them."

In October, again on Dr. Fothergill's advice, Parke set off for Edinburgh to spend the winter in medical studies. To the professors in the northern university he carried introductions from Fothergill and from his old teachers at Philadelphia. He lost no time in delivering his letters; and, cock-sure, noted in his journal his judgement of each. Cullen quite equalled his expectations, greeting him warmly as one recommended by his American friends Morgan and Rush and by Dr. Fothergill, and invited him to call often. Gregory was "quite the Gentleman and indeed much more of the Physician" than Parke expected. He was with Black only a few minutes, yet long enough to convince himself that "he is a good Chemist." The materia medica, he thought, would "gain little improvement" under Home's efforts. Monro, whom he heard lecture, he thought the best orator of all the faculty, but only the third ranking member in point of erudition!

Parke's life at Edinburgh this winter was an uneventful student life. On Cullen's advice he enrolled only in Cullen's course and in Gregory's clinical lectures at the Infirmary. His forenoons were thus filled with formal lectures and the never-ending task of copying notes. The work of making a fair copy of the notes of any single course was onerous. The professors spoke so rapidly that even students with a system of shorthand missed words and phrases. In this situation it was customary for several students to agree literally to compare notes after each lecture; and thus, what one missed another might supply, so that each could have a perfect copy of what the professor said. Parke belonged to such a group and some of the fat volumes of notes he made at Edinburgh bear the notation that they were made by "Thomas Parke and Co." From Cullen alone Parke took upwards of eleven hundred pages of manuscript notes between November and May; and in addition he copied borrowed notes from Cullen's other courses and from Black's.[13] After dinner there was usually a walk and some social visiting. Once a week in the evening lasting until midnight, a student medical society met; from it Parke derived much "improvement."

It was not, of course, all medicine and study at Edinburgh. Parke had time, as his journal records, to read Locke, Robertson's *Charles V,*

[13] These volumes of manuscript notes were presented in 1817 to the library of the Pennsylvania Hospital, where they are preserved.

Humphry Clinker, Hume's *History of England,* and Priestley on electricity, which he borrowed from the University library. He saw a few plays, although he was usually disappointed with them. Parke regularly attended the small Quaker. meeting in Edinburgh; and he was often a guest for tea or supper at the home of William Miller, a great Friend, who took a special interest in the Quaker medical students. Perhaps Parke enjoyed his greatest pleasures with his roommate John Sims. Like him, Sims was a Quaker. They met on the coach travelling to Edinburgh. At first the two found lodging in the same house and later, to save money and out of friendship, they shared a room. Sims was a cheerful and engaging companion to whom Parke gave his confidence without risk of the sort of quarrel that seems to have embittered so many student relations at the University at that time. Together they walked through the city and its environs, made longer jaunts into the country, and went on little excursions with male and female friends; they enjoyed the same quiet pleasures. Sims had Parke to his home in England and when the Philadelphian returned to America, their friendship continued in "an Epistolary way."

Only a few things clouded these pleasant and profitable months at Edinburgh. Parke was occasionally homesick, but letters from home, especially from Owen Biddle, were an infallible cure of this. Parke was ill several times, but his friends cared for him and in his most serious illness Dr. Cullen himself attended him. Most frequently the young student was worried lest he not have enough money to finish his work and live like a gentleman; and there were often periods, especially after a long day of social pleasure, when he reproached himself for not studying harder. But there were nice surprises too: on several occasions, for example, both in London and in Edinburgh, he met Dr. Franklin, who charmed him and drew forth an estimate that he was "certainly as great a Man as America has produced."

In May of 1772 Parke left Edinburgh and proceeded leisurely to London for another season's work in the hospital and another course of lectures. For an hour each morning at seven he attended McKenzie's lectures, then returned home to breakfast and to write until ten or eleven when he went to the Hospital to assist Huck or Fordyce in his work. Yet, because he now knew many people in London, his second stay in the city was fuller of frivolities than his first; he was notably less attentive to his studies. Generally he dined out; often he went to the Pennsylvania Coffee

House in the afternoon for news from Philadelphia and to "hum over" the papers; and scarcely an evening was not filled with some party of pleasure. Of these parties Betsy Corbyn was often a member. Betsy was a charmer and Parke enjoyed her company. He tells in his journal of one high-spirited adventure with Betsy, her sister, and another admirer: "having received information that T.C. and Wife [Betsy's parents] wou'd be out I embraced the opportunity of spending an hour with Betsey—and a happy one it was; found them both more agreeable than ever—Ned Gray also availed himself of the interval, and was happily indulging himself with their company—after conversing as long as we dare stay lest we might be interrupted by the return of Pater and Mater, we decamped a back way highly pleased with our interview and both promised secrecy."

With the coming of winter Parke made his plans to return home. His English friend Robert Barclay, who was heading for America, asked him to join him. In February the two friends carried their baggage aboard the *Pennsylvania Packet,* Captain Osborne; it included a half chest of oranges, some hung beef, and a checker-board. More than two months later, on May 3, the *Pennsylvania Chronicle* published at Philadelphia announced the *Packet's* arrival, carrying, among other persons, "Thomas Parke, M.D." From this time to the end of his life, although he never returned to the College of Philadelphia to take the degree of M.D., he was "Doctor Parke."

Parke was twenty-four when he returned to Philadelphia in the spring of 1773. Welcomed home by his old and ailing preceptor Cadwalader Evans, the younger man was launched at once into practice by the older as his partner. Hardly had Parke begun his work, however, than Dr. Evans died. Three months after his homecoming Thomas Parke thus virtually inherited a very satisfactory practice.[14] He resumed his former friendships, became one of a group of young Quakers who gave themselves romantic names—his was Palemon—and, as he had done in vacations before his trip abroad, occasionally made a pleasure jaunt with them to other places. His innocent flirtations with the lasses of Philadelphia were as gay as with those of London, and his friends chaffed him about them.[15]

Very soon, however, he was seriously interested in Rachel Pemberton,

[14] Parrish, "Thomas Parke," 4-5.
[15] Robert Barclay to Parke, London, Nov. 19, 1774, Barclay Letters, Quaker Collection, Haverford College Library; William Robinson to Parke, New York, July 1, 1774, Society Collection, HSP.

daughter of James Pemberton. The course of true love did not run smoothly for Parke. On his return from a trip to New York—perhaps the lasses there had too evidently attracted him and Rachel had heard about it—he found Miss Rachel cool. Distressed, he wrote his friend Barclay about it, and Barclay offered the despairing lover sage counsel: "My friend dont be disheartened . . . use all diligence to make thy election sure — Women . . . are in their nature suspicious, very much so—the least appearance of coolness awakes every jealousy . . . . I fear ill disposed minds have endeavor'd to proffit by thy absence—fear them not, but by assiduity, care and tenderness endeavor to convince the dear Girl of the perpetuity, reality, and ardor of thy tender regard. . . . thou must work thy own work —to be plain—speak openly, boldly and candidly. the times are critical; press thy suit with ardor . . . ." [16] Probably Thomas followed his friend's advice; at any rate he won Rachel's consent and the engagement was announced late in 1774. The wedding took place the following April. It was an impressive affair as befitted the marriage of a daughter of the Pemberton family. There were several days of dinners and other parties, to which the Quaker aristocracy of the city came in great numbers. Rachel's father spent nearly £500 on his daughter: he provided her with an indentured servant maid, £117 were paid Thomas Affleck for furniture, and not less than £111. 10s. were paid out to Mother Lloyd for "Sundries"—probably Rachel's wardrobe. [17] By his marriage to the grand-daughter of old Israel Pemberton, to a niece of the "King of the Quakers," the young doctor entered into the great world of the Quaker aristocracy. With Evans' practice now largely his and the Pemberton connection to support him, Parke began his career under most favoring circumstances.

Of Parke's practice as a physician there are few records. His conduct, his eulogist declared in 1836, "was marked with more solidity than brilliance—by plain common sense, rather than by the excursive flights of genius." He was "safe and judicious; his opposition to rash and hazardous enterprises might have subjected him to the suspicion of inefficiency in the employment of remedial agents. He knew too well how to estimate the powers of the vis medicatrix naturae, and was not very readily disposed to forsake an old and well tried friend for some new formed acquaintance whose character he did not understand. But when his

[16] Barclay to Parke, New York, June 17, 1774, Barclay Letters.
[17] "Expenditures for Rachel Parke on her marriage," Pemberton Papers, XXVIII, 42. Lists of invited guests are in the same collection, XXVII, 125-127.

judgement led him to employ energetic treatment, he gave ample proof of his ability to conduct it to the benefit of his patient." This essential conservatism was reflected also in his adherence to the conventional pattern of practice which Dr. John Morgan had tried, in vain, to change: Parke dispensed medicines. Toward the sick poor he was "a bright example of kindness and attention"; toward his professional colleagues, whether old or young, he was always mild, dignified, and courteous. Those who knew him in his older age described him as a gentleman of the old school.[18]

In 1777 came a signal testimony to Parke's character and achievement as a man and a physician, as well, no doubt, as to the effect of his Pemberton connection. In May of that year the Managers of the Pennsylvania Hospital elected Parke one of the physicians, in the place of Dr. Morgan who had joined the Continental Army the preceding fall as director-general of the army hospital. They chose him again and again, forty-five times, until he retired at last in 1823.[19] In a life marked by long and devoted service to many institutions of the city, his service to the Pennsylvania Hospital is probably the one for which Parke was best known to his fellow-citizens. In the Hospital as in his private practice Parke was distinguished by no brilliance or originality: he proposed no plans for the care of the sick or the insane; he invented no useful device like John Rhea Barton's hospital bed. But he was regularly in attendance, prescribing for the sick, visiting the insane, giving his advice in consultations; until in time the Hospital became such a part of him and he of it that the Managers had sometimes to remind him of their regulations.

Parke was not a physician of the Hospital a year when Philadelphia was occupied and the British Army took over the Hospital for its own sick and wounded. The Managers attended once a week and Dr. Thomas Bond prescribed for those patients who were kept in the wing the army allowed for civilian use.[20] Parke was still a Hospital physician sixteen years later when a greater crisis overwhelmed the city; one of the doctors who stayed in Philadelphia during the yellow fever epidemic and was stricken by it, he kept his private practice and answered as well the calls of the Hospital Managers in important cases. Of his conduct in these trying days

[18] Parrish, "Thomas Parke," 13.

[19] Thomas G. Morton and Frank Woodbury, *The History of the Pennsylvania Hospital* (Phila. 1895), 563.

[20] Parke to James Pemberton, Phila., Dec. 3, 1777, Pemberton Papers, XXXI, 50.

when the doctors finished a hard day fighting the disease by turning to fight one another on the question of its cause, his eulogist said that he was a peace-maker who tried to preserve harmony between those who followed and those who opposed the theories of Benjamin Rush. Though he failed in his attempt, so convinced were all parties of the unselfishness of his intentions that he preserved the respect of all.[21] To have come through the yellow fever war with reputation unscathed is no small tribute to a physician's character.

Because of Parke's friendships abroad, the Managers frequently asked him to purchase books for the Hospital library, generally from London, sometimes from Hamburg; and when his friend Robert Barclay sent him a sum of money to distribute among worthy American charities Parke chose the Hospital to receive $100 "more especially to the use and comfort of the poor patients in the House." [22] For the insane Parke seems to have had a special concern, as other Quakers had; in 1803 he called on the Managers to forbid indiscriminate visiting of the insane by medical students, as Rush had earlier put a stop to sightseeing by the public; once, too trustful of the insane, Parke gave the freedom of the hospital to a patient who went beserk and attacked another patient; and once Parke himself was stabbed at by a mad woman. One of his patients was the daughter of Luther Martin of Maryland, who particularly asked that the young woman be kept at the Pennsylvania Hospital under Parke's care rather than be sent to a private place.[23]

During Parke's service as physician to the Hospital various proposals were made which would have increased the efficiency and usefulness of the institution and advanced the science of medicine in Philadelphia. While it is hazardous to infer much from a signature added to, or omitted from, a petition, Parke's reaction to these suggestions appears to have been cautious. It was thus in keeping with his character. He did not join Rush, Physick, and Wistar when they called on the Managers to appoint a resident surgeon and he did not sign the petition of Rush, Physick, and Dorsey to appoint two persons to be in charge of the midwifery ward. He

[21] Managers of the Pennsylvania Hospital, Minutes, 10mo. 28, 1793, Pennsylvania Hospital; Parrish, "Thomas Parke," 14-15.

[22] Managers of the Pennsylvania Hospital, Minutes, 5mo. 20, 1799, 10mo. 30, 1815, 2mo. 8, 1816.

[23] *Ibid.*, 5mo. 5, 1800; Morton and Woodbury, *Pennsylvania Hospital,* 141; Martin to Parke, Baltimore, May 20, 26, 1815, Jan. 14, 1816, Etting Papers, Members Old Congress, II, 85, 86, 87, HSP.

opposed the request of the University of Pennsylvania that thirty beds be designated for teaching purposes in the Hospital. On the other hand, he approved granting the presidents of certain learned societies in the city the privilege of the Hospital library; he favored the appointment of a resident apothecary and the erection of a laboratory with a room for the occasional use of the physicians.[24]

On January 27, 1823, Parke submitted his resignation to the Managers. He was seventy-four and age prevented his conveniently performing "the duties of the Station which I have so long endeavoured faithfully to discharge. . . . In reviewing our long and intimate connection," he continued in his formal note of resignation, "I derive much pleasure in the remembrance of the uninterrupted harmony which has accompanied our official intercourse, and though now about to retire from your Board I cherish a hope of retaining a continuance of your individual Esteem." In a postscript he asked the privilege of continuing to visit four private patients, now probably incurable, whose friends and relatives wished them to remain under Parke's care. Accepting the resignation, the Managers spread a brief testimony on their minutes: "The Board cannot part with Doctor Parke who has so long, so faithfully, and so successfully served the Institution without feelings of deep regret and the expression of their solemn wishes for his present and future welfare." [25]

Only a few months after Parke was named a physician of the Pennsylvania Hospital the Quakers of Philadelphia were shocked by the arbitrary arrest of several of their weightiest members whom the Congress and the State Executive Council regarded as inimical to American liberties. They were exiled to Virginia without trial. The spectacle of these prominent Friends being carried through the streets of the very city their grandfathers founded as a haven from persecution must have been profoundly disturbing to each of their co-religionists. Parke was personally involved in the incident because among the Virginia exiles were his father-in-law and two uncles of his wife. He naturally joined with other friends of the unfortunate victims in support of Thomas Mifflin's motion to secure a writ of habeas corpus; but the writ was ignored by the Quakers' guards and the prisoners were carried off all the same. During their relatives' imprisonment Parke and his wife wrote frequently, and Parke made a

[24] Morton and Woodbury, *Pennsylvania Hospital*, 82-84, 457; Pennsylvania Hospital, MS. Archives, 1808, June 23, 1810, March 21, 1820.

[25] Managers of the Pennsylvania Hospital, Minutes, 1st mo. 27, 1823.

midwinter journey to see his father-in-law at Winchester.[26] The bitter
experience of these months made Parke, like other Friends, particularly
receptive to the kind of counsel his friend Barclay offered: ". . . as we pro-
fess principles that lead out of the spirit of the world, let us honestly act
up to them, and not interfere in Public affairs, but keep quiet always
submitting to the powers that are permitted to govern us—."[27]

A year after he was appointed to the staff of the Hospital, in May of
1778, when the British were preparing to evacuate Philadelphia, Parke was
elected a director of the Library Company. When he resigned from the
Board almost fifty-seven years later there was hardly a service he had not
performed for this ancient institution. He was a member of the building
committee and the committee on repairs and improvements; he ordered
books from foreign booksellers; he helped to catalogue the Library's
collection; he often even loaned the Directors money. In the assignments
made to Parke, the meeting of the Directors on May 8, 1794, was typical:
on that day he was named to a committee of correspondence for the im-
portation of foreign books and to a committee for the purchase of American publications; and, with others, he was directed to procure and fix a
lightning rod, have the roof of the Loganian Library painted, and have
the yard north of the Library enclosed. Of only two committees he seems
never to have been a member: those appointed to label the new books and
to come to terms with borrowers who lost books.[28]

He was a member of the committee on foreign purchases for more than
fifty years. His first appointment was in 1782. Three years later he and
Richard Wells were named "a standing Committee to purchase, from
Time to Time, such new Publications as they may think worthy in the
Library." He was given this duty for the last time in 1834, fifty-two years
later. From the Library's agents in England—Joseph Woods and William
Dillwyn in the earlier years of Parke's service—Parke received sales cata-

[26] Parke to James Pemberton, Phila., Sept. 15, 1777; Parke to Pemberton, near
Frederick, Md., Feb. 19, 1778, Pemberton Papers, XXX, 115; XXXI, 142; Parke to
Pemberton, Phila., March 28, 1778, Gilbert Collection of Manuscript Letters, III, 249,
College of Physicians of Philadelphia; Rachel Parke to James Pemberton, Phila., 1st
mo. 28, 1778; Israel Pemberton to Parke, Winchester, 1st mo. 31, 1778, *The Friend,*
LXVIII (1894), 51, 69.
[27] Barclay to Parke, Norwich, Aug. 4, 1778, Barclay Letters.
[28] Directors of the Library Company of Philadelphia, Minutes, May 8, 1794,
passim.

logues; and to them, in his turn, Parke sent the Library's orders on behalf of the Directors. Generally the committee's orders were for specific works: in 1785, for example, Parke's committee ordered thirty-one titles, including Bishop Berkeley's *Principles of Human Knowledge*, Lord Monboddo's *Origin and Progress of Language*, the complete works of Voltaire, Fielding, Richardson, and Johnson, the *Encyclopedia Britannica*, Smyth's *Tour in the United States*, Dobson's *History of the Troubadors*, Bell's *Surgery*, and Swedenborg's works "if to be had in English." Occasionally the instructions were more general, as when Parke in 1789 warned the booksellers to avoid *"Sermons* and medical works—which many of our Constituents think we superabound with, and two Medical Libraries are now forming in this City." [29]

Special tasks were often assigned Parke. When William Bingham expressed a desire to present the new Library Company with a white marble statue, Parke was directed to wait on him to learn his pleasure; and when Bingham announced that his preference was for a statue of Franklin, Parke secured Franklin's approval of the Directors' design that the subject appear in "a Gown for his dress and a Roman head." [30] Parke was one of the committee which a few months later dealt with Samuel Jennings, a former Philadelphian, then a painter in London, who offered the Directors a painting of Clio, Calliope, or Minerva, as they chose. Parke drafted the Directors' reply expressing their preference for Minerva, but suggesting as an alternative "the figure of Liberty (with her Cap and proper Insignia) displaying the arts by some of the most stricking Symbols of Painting, Architecture, Mechanics, Astronomy &c. whilst She appears in the attitude of placing on the top of a Pedestal, a pile of Books, lettered with, *Agriculture, Commerce Philosophy* and *Catalogue of Philadelphia Library*. A Broken Chain under her feet and in the distant back Ground a Groupe of Negroes sitting on the Earth, or in some attitude expressive of Ease and Joy." [31] This suggestion the painter took; and in the Library Company today are preserved both the marble statue of a Roman Franklin and Jennings' painting of Liberty surrounded by her children.

From time to time during the long years of his service Parke presented the Library with books and pamphlets. The list of his gifts is long and varied. The first gift, made the year after his election as a Director, was of

[29] *Ibid.,* Nov. 3. 1785, June 5, 1789.
[30] *Ibid.,* Sept. 3, 1789.
[31] *Ibid.,* May 6, 1790.

the *Trials of Admiral Keppel and Sir Hugh Palliser* and an *Address to Admiral Keppel* by a Seaman; the last gift, made in 1830, seems to have been the second volume of *British Naturalists*. In 1781 Parke gave the Library a copy of Jonathan Carver's *Travels;* in 1784, a collection of pamphlets including sermons, political addresses, and reports of the London Humane Society. On behalf of his friend Barclay he presented several works of travel, including the Proceedings of the Association for Promoting the Discovery of the Interior Parts of Africa. He gave many tracts on slavery and the slave trade. One of his gifts was Mme. de Stael's *Appeal to the Nations of Europe*. Within a few months in 1825 he presented a miscellaneous collection comprising Rev. Mr. R. Bicknell's *The West Indies as they Are*, Rev. B. Dacre's *Testimonies in favor of Salt as a Manure*, James Cropper's *The Present State of Ireland*, Joseph J. Gurney's *Letter on Christianity*, and *Letters on Universal Toleration*. To the Library's natural history cabinet and museum Parke made such gifts as an injected human heart, the dried skin of a loon, a tibia "injected to prove that Bones are Vascular," some English coins, and a silver medal in honor of the Seven Bishops.[32]

In this way, doing these things, for nearly fifty-seven years Parke attended the meetings of the Library Directors regularly. With their formal business the Directors occasionally mixed some pleasures, as a note from Zachariah Poulson, the librarian, to Parke in 1788 reveals: only as much work remained to be done on the catalogue, he explained, as would occupy the Directors until 7 o'clock; "As they mean to devote the Remainder of the Evening to *Oysters* and *social Converse,* they earnestly wish the punctual Attendance of all the Members of the Committee, and have therefore requested ZP. to solicit, in a particular Manner, the Company of Dr. Parke, precisely at *six* o'Clock!" [33]

The first year after his return from England Parke was elected a member of the American Philosophical Society and was at once named to a committee to consider and prepare papers for the second volume of the Society's *Transactions*. For a short time ten years later, he served on the committee to oversee the construction of the Society's building on State House Square; and in 1795 he was elected one of the Society's curators with Charles Willson Peale and Benjamin Smith Barton. But Parke's

[32] *Ibid.,* Aug. 4, 1784, April 27, 1815, Aug. 7, 1823.
[33] *Ibid.,* Nov. 19, 1788.

interests and accomplishments were not like those of the most active philosophers; he must have found little pleasure or satisfaction in their meetings, for he attended infrequently—between 1806 and 1815 he was present only once—and in 1817 he submitted his resignation. Although this was not laid before the Society and therefore not accepted, he never attended another meeting of the Society.[34]

Yet Parke cannot be said to have been entirely uninterested in science. Like so many other Quakers and physicians of the eighteenth century, like Peter Collinson and Alexander Garden, for examples, Thomas Parke was interested in natural history, especially in botany. This interest, to be sure, was not that of an original investigator, for Parke never described a new specimen; he seems never to have reflected or speculated on botanical matters or even to have taken a botanizing trip. His interest was rather that of the gentleman amateur, friend and patron of botanists. Although Dr. John Coakley Lettsom thought Parke might become the center of a natural history society in Philadelphia, perhaps Parke's most useful role in botany was as the American agent for Humphry Marshall, his onetime Chester County neighbor. Marshall, like John Bartram, a self-taught botanist, kept a nursery at Marshallton, Pennsylvania, where he sold American trees, shrubs, plants and seeds, especially to the gardens of England. The trade in American herbs for their medicinal properties was long established; now, however, the gentlemen of England were interested in gardening as a hobby; they vied with one another to decorate their country places with exotics imported from around half the world. They especially coveted American specimens. Humphry Marshall was one of those who supplied these specimens, and almost all his correspondence on the subject passed through Thomas Parke.

As early as 1771 when he left Philadelphia for his London studies, young Parke offered to carry letters or perform any commissions in England and Scotland with which Marshall would entrust him. Marshall asked two things, that Parke recommend him to English seedsmen and that he look up his Derbyshire forebears, although in neither business did Parke meet with much success. Meanwhile in London Dr. Fothergill occasionally asked Parke to perform some errand in the line of natural history. Once he sent the young man to the docks to pick up a snake

[34] Parke to John Vaughan, Phila., July 12, 1817, MS. Archives, American Philosophical Society; Henry Phillips, Jr., *Early Proceedings of the American Philosophical Society* (Phila., 1884), 87, 154, 227, *passim*.

skin consigned to him; but the customs officials were doubtful whether to admit it—a piece of bureaucratic stupidity from which Parke persuaded them, "as the snake, if entire and alive, would do no harm to the nation, and certainly the skin cannot."[35]

The association of Parke and Marshall grew closer after the former's return from England. For example, Marshall asked Parke's advice on the medical education of his nephew Moses; Parke replied recommending a winter in Philadelphia in the study of anatomy and chemistry and attendance on the practice of the Pennsylvania Hospital. However, he admitted the expense would be great, and there was no likelihood of a job for Moses except possibly as assistant apothecary at the Hospital. A few years later when Moses Marshall wanted to undertake a botanical trip to Kentucky, Parke sought, unsuccessfully as it proved, the financial assistance of the American Philosophical Society.[36]

The resumption of normal trade with England after the Revolution permitted Marshall's seed business to grow and, since Dr. Parke was Marshall's designated American agent and most of the correspondence passed through him, Parke's work was increased as well. One of Marshall's most regular English customers was Parke's good friend Robert Barclay. He was now a prospering London merchant, soon to be part owner of Thrale's brewery which he would improve with a steam engine made by Boulton and Watt and from which he would frequently send hampers of beer to his Philadelphia friend.[37] (This association of Dr. Parke with Barclay and thus, albeit slightly, with Dr. Samuel Johnson's circle and with James Watt is an interesting commentary on the size of the eighteenth-century world.) From lists which Marshall prepared and Parke transmitted to England and from Marshall's botanical catalogue *Arbustrum Americanum,* published in 1785, Barclay selected specimens to plant in his own garden and to present as gifts for the gardens of his friends. Occasionally he asked Parke (and Parke relayed some of the requests to Marshall) for something for his cabinet—once it was some new American coins, maps, and prints of leading characters; then it was "two fine mock-

[35] William Darlington, *Memorials of John Bartram and Humphry Marshall* (Philadelphia, 1849), 523-527; Fothergill to Parke, [London, Nov.] 30, [1772], Pemberton Papers, XXXIV, 167.

[36] Darlington, *Memorials,* 527, 528.

[37] James L. Clifford, *Hester Lynch Piozzi (Mrs. Thrale)* (Oxford, 1941), 201-202; Barclay to Parke, London, Feb. 7, 1787, Barclay Letters.

ing birds" and some dried humming birds; again it was some live par-
tridges and, if possible, live pheasants, which he meant to give to his
Norfolk neighbor Lord Suffield. When Suffield himself became a cus-
tomer Barclay sent Parke detailed instructions how to handle this distinguished account: specifically, Marshall's letters must be copied by
Moses, as the older man's untrained hand would make a bad impression
on the nobleman. Sir Joseph Banks, president of the Royal Society, bought
plants of Marshall, and so did Sir John Menzies who wanted seeds of
American forest trees and some American fruit trees for the place in
Scotland which he was planting. From these customers Marshall generally received payment in the form of medicines and chemicals, books,
and instruments. In 1787 a more business-like relation opened when Grimwood, Hudson and Barrit, nursery-owners and seedsmen of London,
through Dr. Parke, began a correspondence with Marshall.[38]

Nearer home, Parke and Marshall were both close to William Hamilton when he planned and planted the gardens at Woodlands, near Philadelphia. It was Parke who introduced Marshall and Hamilton, thus
inaugurating a long friendship between the seedsman and the gentleman
botanist; and it was Parke to whom Hamilton committed a number of
responsibilities in connection with his estate and his family during his
absence from America. When Hamilton went abroad in 1784 he named
Parke and Edward Shippen his attorneys and during the two years of
his absence he showered both men with instructions as well as with travel
accounts. Seeing the country places of England, he conceived the plan of
making his new home at Woodlands the model of an English estate and
bent his energies to this end. When Hamilton heard of the death of the
botanist William Young, he directed Parke to buy Young's potted plants
or, if the widow would not sell at once, to persuade her to do nothing
until he could see her. He engaged several stone quarriers in England and
sent them to Philadelphia with instructions to Parke to put them to work
at Woodlands. Complaining of the high cost of living in England and his
own lack of funds, he asked the obliging doctor to send him some cured
beef, apples, nuts, and roasting ears from the estate.[39] Sometimes Hamilton

[38] Darlington, *Memorials,* 530-532; Barclay to Parke, London, Feb. 7, 1787,
July 18, 1788; Norwich, Sept. 28, 1788; London, Dec. 3, 1789, Barclay Letters; Parke
to Marshall, Phila., Aug. 6, 1785; Grimwood, Hudson & Barrit to Marshall, London,
Feb. 6, 1787, Humphry Marshall Correspondence, I, 20, 35, Dreer Collection, HSP.
[39] Darlington, *Memorials,* 528; Sarah P. Stetson, "William Hamilton and his

asked Parke to perform services of a more delicate nature. Now Parke must see to it that Molly, Hamilton's ward, was put at once to the harpsichord and pianoforte and then sent to a dancing master; now he must do something about Mrs. Hamilton's "arrant nonsense" in refusing to allow Peggy to go out in public parties for want of a proper person to introduce her. It is pleasant to record that these services were appreciated: Ann Hamilton sent him a goblet with "hopes he will enjoy many Draughts of porter out of it"; and William Hamilton, directing Parke to have the ice house at Bush Hill filled before his return, promised the doctor that they would then "crack a *cool* Bottle" together with old friends.[40]

Another of Parke's botanical friends was John Coakley Lettsom. This prominent Quaker physician, who succeeded Fothergill in a fashionable and extensive London practice, bought seeds and plants for his garden. Thanks to Marshall, he wrote Parke, he had "a tolerably good collection of American plants, though young." Ever an enthusiast for natural history as for all good works, he encouraged Parke to take the lead in an American society of natural history. Science and the national economy, he urged, both called for it. "Your extensive Country which almost includes both Zones is capable of nourishing all the productions nearly of the Globe. It would afford an useful employment for patriots of leisure and Science, to form Societies, and promote the introduction of Exotics, that tend to utility or pleasure. Why may not South Carolina export Tea, and Philadelphia Rhubarb?—You abound in Timber, but Mahogany, and various other things might thrive on your Mountains, whilst feebler exotics might enrich your Vallies—Such as Grapes of different kinds—Olives and Mulberries—

"These are studies," Lettsom continued, "which appear to me more patriotic than hanging Loyalists and more worthy of an enlightened people than expelling an industrious but unfortunate race—Perhaps I am wrong in my Sentiments, but I have always thot with the persian Conqueror

---

'Woodlands,'" *Pennsylvania Magazine of History and Biography,* LXXIII (1949), 26-33; Barclay to Parke, London, Nov. 6, 1782, Barclay Letters; Hamilton to Parke, London, Aug. 22, 1785, Society Collection, HSP; Hamilton, Power of Attorney, Phila., Oct. 2, 1784, Gratz Collection, Provincial Conference 1776, HSP.

[40] Hamilton to Parke, London, Sept. 25, Nov. 2, 1785, Dreer Collection; Ann Hamilton to Parke, n.p., n.d., Charles Roberts Autograph Collection, Haverford College Library.

> Ils sont hommes comme nous, ils ne sont plus
> ennemis, sitôt qu'ils sont vaincus.

I doubt not however, but my frd Parke as an individual will join in these sentiments of Cyrus . . . ."[41]

Two years later, writing to Marshall, Lettsom spoke encouragingly of a society of natural history recently gathered in London. "Such a Society, established in Philadelphia, might be very important. A man of Dr. Parke's influence, with very few others to begin it, would excite emulation in your citizens, and give vigour and permanency to such an institution." The next year he returned to his theme in a letter to Parke: there ought to be societies of natural history and mineralogy in America "to bring to light the treasures you possess." America was greatly endowed with natural riches but did not know its own wealth. Half the wealth of England rested on one article alone; and America possessed coal too. "Why do you not open this mine, which exposes itself upon the banks of many of your rivers?" American gums, dyewoods, and medicinal plants were numerous. "Why don't you discover and ascertain them?" Lettsom concluded with an appeal to Parke and all enlightened Americans: "Try to commence these Societies—perhaps the English are not such enemies to you, but there might be Individuals to aid your endeavours." [42]

But Dr. Parke never responded to Lettsom's appeals. Although it appears he planned an herbarium, no natural history society was ever founded through his efforts or even with his encouragement. To the end of his life Parke was interested in his garden and had a gardener who supplied it; but other men founded the Academy of Natural Sciences in 1816 and Parke was never a member.[43]

Meanwhile his wife Rachel bore him five children, of whom two died young. In the records are occasional glimpses of the young married couple making a little trip together, once "over the stony and mountainous Land of the Wilderness" to the romantic Susquehanna, where they called on the famous female poet Lucy Wright and returned via Lancaster, Ephrata, Reading, and Bethlehem. In another letter the proud and loving father speaks of "our lovely little Boy" whose "winning playfull Smile" was such

[41] Lettsom to Parke, London, July 21, 1785, Etting Papers, Scientists, 56.

[42] Darlington, *Memorials,* 545: Lettsom to Parke, London, Aug. 1788, Gilbert Collection of MS. Letters, III, 65.

[43] Lettsom to Parke, London, Feb. 3, 1789, Etting Papers, Scientists, 57.

a joy to his parents.[44] But Mrs. Parke was never robust or well. There are several references to an indisposition. Her trouble was a consumption, which sapped her strength and after fourteen weeks' confinement to bed killed her in March 1786 at the early age of thirty-two. She was buried, her father wrote his brother, on March 11, "with becoming solemnity and exemplary decency." The shock of her death, James Pemberton continued, was "a disposition of close exercise to her husband, with whom she maintained a strict affection . . . ."[45]

After Rachel Parke's death Dr. Parke's life seems to reveal a new color. It is possible that event was the cause, by loosening the ties which bound Parke closely to the Pemberton family and thus kept him closely under the strict discipline of the Society of Friends. But, whatever the cause, it is remarkable and interesting that the same Thomas Parke who signed the Quakers' petition against the stage in 1783 was a guest for dinner at the home of Thomas Wignell less than twenty years later. It is, of course, true that though he was a serious youth, Parke was never a solemn sobersides. He had a genius for friendship and a talent for serving his friends, as Jacob Duché and Phineas Bond and other unhappy victims of the Revolution testified. He was always an agreeable companion; as a young man he had always a keen, appraising eye for beauty in the other sex. But in the last fifteen years of the century, after his wife's death, Parke developed into that most attractive type, the gay and social Friend beloved by youth and age alike. He was never without an invitation for dinner, cards, or social chat. Indeed half the surviving Parke manuscripts are social invitations. He was often at William Hamilton's of course, and at John Penn's, who was his patient as well as his friend. There is an invitation to tea in 1787 from "Mr Pine and all the Females of his Family," and an invitation to dinner in 1818 from the Count Survilliers, formerly Joseph Bonaparte, king of Spain. Josiah Hewes asked him "to attend . . . the Dissection of a Codfish—Dinner"; and Miss Ellen Lyle promised "peasoup, strawberries and cream at half past two precisely." Parke went frequently to Miss Bond's for cards; and notes on each printed

[44] Parke to Sally and Hannah Pemberton, Susquehanna River, [1778?], Pemberton Papers, XXXII, 150; Parke to Hannah Pemberton, Phila., Aug. 21, 1780, Etting Papers, Physicians, 72.
[45] James Pemberton to John Pemberton, 3mo. 18, 1786, in John and Isaac Comly, eds., *Friends' Miscellany* . . . (Phila., 1835), VII, 78-79; Hinshaw, *Encyclopedia*, II, 402.

invitation indicate the number of guests present—now fifty, now eighty, now a hundred. He belonged to a gentlemen's club called the Catch, where one paid half a dollar each evening on entrance "(for your Liquor)." [46]

When he died in 1835 Thomas Parke was president of the College of Physicians of Philadelphia. He had held that office since 1818; he had been a member of the College since its inception in 1787 and was its last surviving founder. Dr. Rush had been most active in originating and organizing the College; as one of the older physicians in the city Parke had been invited to join. As the constitution of the College put it simply, the purposes of the association were "to advance the Science of Medicine, and thereby to lessen Human Misery, by investigating the diseases and remedies which are peculiar to our Country, by observing the effects of different seasons, climates, and situations upon the Human body, by recording the changes that are produced in diseases by the progress of Agriculture, Arts, Population, and Manners, by searching for Medicines in our Woods, Waters, and the bowels of the Earth, by enlarging our avenues to knowledge; from the discoveries and publications of foreign Countries; by appointing stated times for Literary intercourse and communications, and by cultivating uniformity and order in the practice of Physick." [47]

These ideas were expressed in the activities of the College and in the work Dr. Parke was called on to do. He was often particularly charged with library affairs. On March 3, 1789, he was named a member of the library committee, which was instructed to purchase books; and a few months later he was elected one of the censors, whose duties included the oversight of the library. As he so often did for the Library Company, so

[46] Many of these social notes are in the Etting Collection, HSP; others are in the possession of Dr. Thomas Parke, a collateral descendant, of Downingtown, Pa., to whom I wish to express my thanks for allowing me to see them. Dr. Parke's collection provided the materials for an interesting newspaper article entitled "Echoes of Philadelphia in colonial days. Dr. Parke's treasured cards of invitation recall social gatherings of olden time celebrities," published in the Philadelphia *Public Ledger,* April 8, 1906. The Quaker memorial against the theater is in Revolutionary Papers, XLV, 10, Archives Division, Pennsylvania State Historical and Museum Commission, Harrisburg.

[47] W. S. W. Ruschenberger, *An Account of the institution and progress of the College of Physicians of Philadelphia* (Phila., 1887), 175.

for the College of Physicians Parke purchased books abroad. The sums the College had to spend on its library were necessarily limited; but the committee's buying showed an intelligent policy of purchasing the important series like the *Memoirs* of the London Medical Society, the Leipzig *Commentaries, the Mémoires* of the Académie royale de Chirurgie, and the *Edinburgh Medical and Surgical Journal,* as well as single works like those of Monro and Lieutaud's *Synopsis Medica.* In 1818, the year he was elected president, Parke was one of the committee which prepared a catalogue of the library, a task which was performed in a neat and accurate manner to the entire satisfaction of the Fellows.[48]

The preparation of a national pharmacopoeia was a project of the medical profession inspired by national pride and the actual necessities of American practice. As early as 1789 the College appointed a committee on the subject, which published an address to "the most respectable medical characters in the United States," asking for their cooperation in preparing such a volume. Nothing came of this call, but the committee continued in existence and Parke was added to it in 1794. Some years later the Massachusetts Medical Society produced a pharmacopoeia, and in 1818 the Medical Society of the State of New York revived the idea of a national work. Regional meetings preceded the national meeting at Washington; Dr. Parke presided over the middle states meeting which gathered in the hall of the College of Physicians at Philadelphia in 1819, and he was one of the delegates from this regional convention to the national meeting which finally prepared and approved a pharmacopoeia. Although in some particulars the final work differed from the plan of the middle states, Parke heartily endorsed it. When a revised edition appeared in 1832, he signed the paper of the College of Physicians recommending its use to all physicians.[49]

Even in his own specialty of medicine, Thomas Parke was not an original thinker. Unlike Rush, who was usually so full of ideas that he had to write to give himself relief, Parke was the author of little. He was, however, one of the committee of the College which drew up a statement on the yellow fever as it had appeared in 1793 and 1797, with an account of the best methods of preventing its introduction into the city in the future. To the College he read one paper on the uses of arsenic in rheu-

[48] College of Physicians, Minutes, July 5, 1791, Feb. 5, 1793, June 2, 1795, July 7, 1818, Jan. 5, 1819.
[49] Ruschenberger, *College of Physicians,* 101-114.

matism which was later deemed worthy of publication. And when in 1827 the College proposed that at each of its meetings a Fellow read a learned paper, Parke presented one on the uses of cold and warm bathing. But when his turn came up two years later, he begged to be excused and sent in his forfeit of one dollar.[50]

The contributions of voluntary associations like the College of Physicians have been insufficiently comprehended; many community responsibilities were discharged, and often adequately, by organizations unknown to the law. In Philadelphia the College of Physicians often served as a kind of advisory public health office; sometimes it gave its opinions on its own initiative, often it prepared them in response to a specific request from the mayor of the city or the governor of the commonwealth. Parke was one of those who in 1793 prepared the answers to a series of questions propounded by Governor Mifflin on the nature of yellow fever and the possible defenses against it. With Dr. Rush and Dr. John Jones he drafted a petition to the House of Representatives of the new republic in 1790 urging that the excessive use of spirituous liquors be curbed. He proposed plans to the Board of Health on behalf of the College in 1795 for the construction of a hospital for contagious diseases. And when the state legislature in 1794 proposed to regulate the practice of medicine, the College made representations and rewrote the legislative proposals to make them more consistent with the actual conditions of medical practice in Pennsylvania.[51] All these are significant public services.

Such a public service, one of the most unusual Dr. Parke performed, was the interest of the College of Physicians in the Zimmerman case. On December 7, 1824, Dr. Joseph Parrish reported to the College that one John Zimmerman was then under sentence of death in the Schuylkill County prison, but that there was evidence of his insanity at the time he committed the crime. A committee to investigate was appointed; acting swiftly, it satisfied itself of the facts and only two days later produced a memorial to the governor asking a reprieve. Governor Schulze welcomed the memorial, granted the reprieve, had Zimmerman examined by a local committee of physicians, and when they disagreed, said he should like to have the opinion of "some of the intelligent Physicians of Philadelphia on this perplexing case. Under the Law of Pennsylvania the executive has no

[50] College of Physicians, Minutes, Dec. 11, 1798, Oct. 4, 1808, April 3, 1827, July 3, 1827, Oct. 24, 1829.
[51] Ibid., Dec. 7, 1790, Nov. 19, 1793, March 10, 14, 1794, Feb. 10, 1795.

other means of obtaining the necessary information, there being no mode but that which arises from the humanity of our citizens." Another committee from the College was accordingly appointed; Parke was on it. And although he was at this time more than seventy-five years old Parke travelled from Philadelphia to Pottstown to examine Zimmerman and submit a report to the governor.[52]

Old age was now coming fast upon him. In 1823 Parke had resigned his post as a physician of the Pennsylvania Hospital. After 1830 his attendance on the meetings of the College of Physicians became less regular and, accordingly, at the end of that year, he submitted his resignation both as a Fellow and as president. This resignation became an annual affair. Each year, when it was received, the College would appoint a committee to wait upon Parke and ask him to withdraw it, and each year the committee reported back that their old president was moved to resign only because he feared could no longer perform the duties of his office. After 1831 he was never again present in the College of Physicians. His illness was a stroke which left one leg paralyzed and affected his mind slightly; old friends meeting him on the street grieved to see tears fill his eyes as, pointing to his useless leg, he tried to tell them what had happened. His memory failed; staring vacantly, talking to unseen friends, he imagined sometimes that he was travelling and in his own house demanded to know the tariff. At night there were some frightening scenes when Parke, thinking himself again at the Hospital, went stamping about crying for the senior pupil.[53]

He died on January 9, 1835, at his house in Locust Street where he had lived with his children to care for him. Formal printed funeral invitations were sent to 228 persons—the list was as carefully preserved as the list of guests at his wedding sixty years before. Most of the medical faculty came, all the older men who had been his colleagues, and many of the younger whom he had welcomed into the fellowship of the profession; some of his Quaker relations, friends of long standing whom he had met over the dinner tables at Woodlands and Lansdowne so long ago. The old names

---

[52] Ruschenberger, *College of Physicians*, 120-123; John Andrew Schulze to Parke, Harrisburg, Jan. 17, Feb. 28, 1825; George M. Stroud to Joseph Parrish, Harrisburg, March 16, March 19, 1825, College of Physicians, MS. Archives, 569, 573, 577, 579.
[53] Parrish, "Thomas Parke," 16-17; College of Physicians, Minutes, Nov. 30, 1830, Jan. 31, 1832, Aug. 27, 1833, Feb. 25, 1834.

were there, like Deborah Logan and Sarah Wistar, Benjamin Chew and Cadwalader Evans, Clement Biddle and Bishop White; and the newer names, now growing familiar too, of Alexander Wilson, Dr. Horner, Dr. George B. Wood, Robert Hare, and Thomas T. Hewson, son of that Dr. William Hewson of London to whom he had borne letters of introduction, the man who would succeed him as president of the College of Physicians.[54]

Solidity rather than brilliance; plain common sense rather than the flights of genius—this, said his eulogist before the College the next year, was the mark of the man's character. Parke had participated in many of the city's activities, though he had originated none and been a leader in few. Yet he served his place and time well by serving them as he could, honestly, industriously, faithfully. Nothing was worse for his having lived, much was a bit better. These are not indifferent talents, or this a negligible achievement. They are the talents and achievements, the strength as they are perhaps the weakness, of a democratic society.

[54] Etting Papers, Miscellaneous, II, 128, 130. By the terms of his will Dr. Parke left his house in Locust Street to his children, none of whom had married; and to each of them he bequeathed in addition some stocks and bonds. Thomas, who had been a merchant travelling to India, received his father's cane and the desk which Dr. Parke had inherited from *his* father. There were small bequests to a niece and two friends and to several charities. The Library Company and the Pennsylvania Hospital each received some ground rents. Thomas Parke, "Will," Aug. 15, 1828, Will Book, XI, 375, Register of Wills, Philadelphia.

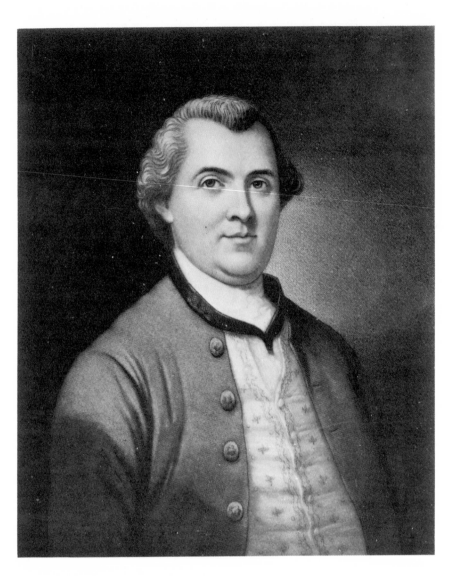

JAMES HUTCHINSON

JAMES HUTCHINSON (1752–1793):
A PHYSICIAN IN POLITICS

THE HISTORY OF THE FOUNDING AND OF THE EARLY YEARS OF THE FIRST medical school in British North America has been often and fully told. The outstanding members of the first faculty have found biographers, and the principal associated institutions, such as the Pennsylvania Hospital and the College of Physicians, have had their historians. The second generation of medical professors has not fared so well, nor is so much known about medical education and the nature of the profession in the fifteen years between the outbreak of the American Revolution and the reorganization of the Medical School of the University of Pennsylvania in 1791. In contrast to Rush, Shippen, Morgan, and even Kuhn, we know almost nothing about the lives and work of Benjamin Smith Barton, John Carson, Samuel P. Griffitts, Thomas C. James, Caspar Wistar, and others. One of these little-known figures is James Hutchinson, professor of chemistry and materia medica in the University of the State of Pennsylvania, 1789–91, and of chemistry in the University of Pennsylvania, 1791–93.

Hutchinson was born in Makefield Township, Bucks County, Pennsylvania, on January 29, 1752, the second child but first son of Randall Hutchinson, a stonemason, and Catherine Rickey, his second wife, both plain country Friends.[1] The elder Hutchinson was something of a local character—Alexander Graydon's family recalled him as a "queer put"—who used to entertain his workmen after the day's work with verses sung "in rustic drone." A favorite was a satire on the aristocratic party of the day entitled "An Attempt

---

[1] James Thacher, *American Medical Biography* (Boston, 1828), 1: 309–11; *Dictionary of American Biography*; Randall Hutchinson, Will, dated November 8, 1760, Will Book No. 3, p. 41, Register of Wills, Bucks Co., Pa.; *Pennsylvania Archives*, 2nd ser., 9: 238 (hereafter cited as *Pa. Archives*).

to Wash the Black-Moor White."[2] Though it is doubtful that Randall Hutchinson could have influenced his son's thinking, for he died when the lad was nine, it is nonetheless true that James's political views were like his father's, critical and democratic.

James went first to a neighborhood school kept by Paul Preston, a successful teacher with a growing reputation, whom admirers denominated "a self-taught genius"; he is said to have been sent thereafter to an academy in Burlington, New Jersey, and then to a school in Virginia, possibly in Alexandria. Perhaps some responsibility for the boy's education had already been assumed by Israel Pemberton, the wealthy Philadelphia merchant and one of the weightiest Friends in the Yearly Meeting, who was a friend or even remote relation of the family, and whom James called "uncle." Pemberton, or another, apprenticed the lad, then about fifteen years of age, to the Philadelphia Quaker apothecaries Moses and Isaac Bartram; James remained with them four years. He attended the shop and "Elaboratory," prepared drugs and compounded prescriptions, read at least a few medical texts, sometimes accompanied his masters on calls to the sick, and generally acquired not only book knowledge of botany, chemistry, and pharmacy but also some understanding of medical practice.

So promising did the lad appear that early in 1771 his stepfather (Catherine Hutchinson had remarried) or Pemberton apprenticed him to Cadwalader Evans, a Quaker physician who enjoyed a good reputation and a profitable practice in Philadelphia and was one of the physicians to the Pennsylvania Hospital. While he was Evans' apprentice, Hutchinson registered for medical lectures at the College of Philadelphia and also for the private lectures on natural philosophy delivered by Christopher Colles.[3]

In the late winter of 1772, however, Hutchinson's studies were interrupted. Pemberton's son Charles was seriously ill, probably with tuberculosis. The local doctors prescribed a sea voyage, and Pemberton asked his young protégé to accompany the ailing son to Barbados. Charles seemed to gain strength on the trip, but he began to hemorrhage again just as the vessel

[2] Alexander Graydon, *Memoirs of His Own Time* (Philadelphia, 1846), pp. 91–92. The verses attacked Judge William Moore and others of the Proprietary party, including Dr. Thomas Bond, and praised Benjamin Franklin, Isaac Norris, and Joseph Galloway as patriots devoted to the cause of liberty; a copy is in the Library Company of Philadelphia.
[3] Hutchinson's tickets of admission to the lectures are in the Hutchinson Papers, American Philosophical Society Library, Philadelphia, Pa.

reached Bridgetown; two weeks later he died. "I set up with him the last six Nights of his Illness," Hutchinson reported; but nothing had availed.[4]

In the spring of 1773 the apothecary of the Pennsylvania Hospital resigned his post. With the encouragement of his preceptor Dr. Evans and with recommendations from his professor Benjamin Rush and from Isaac Bartram, who wrote that he was "fully Capable of Conducting any one of the Processes in the Pharmaceutic Parts of Chymistry," Hutchinson applied for the appointment, as did another student. The committee which examined the candidates concluded that both were qualified but observed that "the Interest of the Hospital will be promoted by the Choice of him whose future Prospect in Life renders him the most likely to continue the greatest Length of Time in that Station." Apparently Hutchinson was prepared to stay longer than his rival, for he received the appointment; and on May 17, 1773, he began his duties. He prepared lists of drugs, compounded prescriptions, kept records of students attending the Hospital practice, and gave instruction to Jacob Ehrenzellar, who was apprenticed to the Hospital in June, 1773, to learn the trade of pharmacy. His salary was fixed at £70 annually.[5]

It was probably because his formal education had been interrupted, first by the trip to Barbados as Charles Pemberton's medical attendant, then by his duties as Hospital apothecary, that Hutchinson did not receive the degree of bachelor of medicine from the College until 1774. No public commencement was held that year, because of the troubled political situation, and he received his diploma, dated August 1, in private. At the same time the Trustees awarded him a gold medal for excellence in chemistry. On one side his name and the date were engraved; on the other, the Latin sentiment,

[4] Hutchinson to Pemberton, 2 mo. 23, April 12, 1772, Pemberton Papers, 23: 85, 111, Historical Society of Pennsylvania; Hutchinson to Pemberton, 3 mo. 30, 1772, Charles Roberts Autograph Collection, Haverford College Library, Haverford, Pa.

[5] Thomas G. Morton and Frank Woodbury, *The History of the Pennsylvania Hospital, 1751–1895* (Philadelphia, 1895), p. 532; Pennsylvania Hospital Managers, Minutes, May 8, 31, June 26, 1773, June 26, 1775; certificates to the Hospital Managers by Isaac Bartram, Cadwalader Evans, and Benjamin Rush, Hutchinson Papers; except where otherwise noted, all manuscripts cited below are in the Hutchinson Papers in the American Philosophical Society Library. Soon afterward Rush and Hutchinson fell out: in the Hutchinson Papers is an undated fragment in which the latter protests Rush's publication of an attack on something he had written, as "a harsh and unjust attempt, not merely to check the inoffensive ambition of a Young man, but if possible to embarrass and defeat him in his entrance upon the duties of an Arduous Profession." The two men were never reconciled.

Naturae artique arcana retexi—"I have discovered the mysteries of nature and of art."[6]

Thus by 1774 James Hutchinson had acquired about as much formal medi-cal training and experience as a young man could expect to get in the Ameri-can colonies at that time. He might have settled in Philadelphia or one of the neighboring towns and practiced with credit and profit. But, if he ex-pected to rank in the profession with his teachers Rush and Shippen, or with his friend Thomas Parke, he must go abroad for more training. Apparently he could expect nothing from his stepfather, but was dependent upon the interest and generosity of Israel Pemberton. He remained another year at the Hospital as its apothecary.

Philadelphia in the winter of 1774–75 was an exciting, disturbing place. The meeting of the first Continental Congress, the closing of the port of Boston, the effects of the Non-Importation Agreement, and military prepara-tions and alarms were unsettling for all, but especially for a country Quaker. Hutchinson knew he was supposed to be peaceful and neutral and loyal; but he was also moved in an unquakerly way by the appeals and deeds of his countrymen and of those whom he began to regard as his country's enemies. Israel Pemberton watched the young man's responses with growing appre-hension, then decided on a course of action which would both keep him from political distractions and promote his professional advancement. He offered to pay for a year's study in London.

The combination of sound training as an apprentice and a student at the College with practical experience as the Hospital apothecary had prepared Hutchinson well for the kind of professional education London offered. In addition, he carried excellent personal introductions to the solid, prosperous, influential Quaker society of the capital, particularly to Dr. John Fothergill, friend and correspondent of Israel Pemberton, one of the busiest and best-known London practitioners, who took a special interest in everyone from Pennsylvania.

The voyage was swift and uneventful, except that the ship passed an ice-berg—a surprising sight to a Philadelphian in July. Disembarking at King-road in the mouth of the Avon, Hutchinson traveled up to Bristol, where he lingered three days with friends and visited the principal local sights, among them Gabriel Goldney's garden and grotto, with its exhibit of fossils and other natural curiosities, an artificial waterfall, and a goldfish pond. These

[6] University of Pennsylvania *Alumni Register*, 4, no. 7 (mid-March, 1900): 8–10.

pleased him; but, remembering that he had come to England for serious things, he hastily assured his uncle that had they not been on his route, he would "not have lost any time, or been at any expence in seeing them, being detirmined through divine assistance to pay no attention to any other object than improvement in Medical Knowledge." To make up for dawdling in Bristol, he traveled almost nonstop to London, a fifteen-hour journey that left barely enough time to identify the towns and villages the post chaise flew through.[7]

Dr. Fothergill was still in the country. Until he should return, Hutchinson busied himself with presenting his other letters and with informally attending the Aldersgate Dispensary, where young Dr. John Coakley Lettsom introduced him.[8] Because most of the American medical students in Britain in the preceding fifteen years had scorned surgery, Fothergill strongly urged Hutchinson to prepare himself in that specialty and advised him to register as a pupil of Percivall Pott's at St. Bartholomew's Hospital. Though appalled at Pott's 50-guinea fee, Hutchinson felt that he had to take Fothergill's advice and, hoping Uncle Pemberton would understand, bought a ticket on October 3, 1775. On Fothergill's advice he enrolled also for the lectures and dissections of Dr. William Hunter and for Mr. John Hunter's lectures on surgery and comparative anatomy.

"I have the greatest Prospects of improvement in Surgery," he wrote his uncle on December 20.

I have great Opportunities, and great advantages. The Professors take me by the Hand, and the Surgeons of eminence are all kind to me. I dress daily at the Hospital, and am often permitted to perform some of the less Capital Operations myself, and generally assist in the performing of the more Capital ones. This distinction I owe in a great degree to the kindness of Surgeon Pott. In fine should my endeavours be blessed by providence with success, and should I live to return to my native land, I am flattered by my friends that I shall sometime be capable of delivering a Course of Lectures on this very important Branch of Medicine. This at present however is only *Ideal*, and I would not wish my *Medical Friends* in Philadelphia to know that I had even an *Idea* of such a thing. A person capable of this is much wanted in Philadelphia; for such there is a good vacancy, and as I am so happy to stand well with the Pupils, there will be no harm in endeavouring to be qualified for such an undertaking. But tho' my attention is principally directed to Surgery and Midwifery, yet I by no means neglect Physic. I wish for improvement in every part of the Healing Art. I wish to be able to expel the raging Fever, to make diseases die.

[7] Hutchinson to Pemberton, 8 mo. 30, 1775.
[8] Lettsom to Thomas Parke, September 10, 1775.

Within a few weeks of coming to London, he was convinced of the city's incomparable professional advantages. Though medicine, he assured his friends, was taught better at the College of Philadelphia than in London, London excelled in surgery, because it had more patients, more cadavers for study, and more and better teachers. "To that branch of the healing Art my attention has as yet been entirely devoted." Pott, he continued, was eminent for "Judicious Practical Observations," John Hunter for theoretical knowledge and "indefatigable industry in investigating the hitherto concealed laws of the Animal Oeconomy," while Dr. William Hunter was thought to be probably "the best Anatomist now living, and . . . perhaps the best Physiologist."[9]

In the spring term, still taking Fothergill's advice, Hutchinson attended lectures on chemistry, materia medica, and practice delivered by the tireless Dr. George Fordyce, physician to St. Thomas's Hospital, from 7 o'clock to 10 o'clock each morning. In addition, he heard lectures on midwifery by Dr. Thomas Denman, physician and accoucheur of Middlesex Hospital. Someone gave him a ticket to the lectures on botany by William Curtis, an agreeable young Quaker physician, but he could not afford the price of a course on natural history and natural philosophy. Throughout the year he continued his attendance at Bart's and, thanks to his being a student of Fordyce and Denman, could also witness the principal operations at other hospitals. Hutchinson had reason to be satisfied with his work, for, as he wrote Pemberton, he was taken notice of by men of science and was elected a member of one or two "literary" societies.[10]

Though grateful to be in England—"this Island, where science dwells"— Hutchinson did not especially like London, which he found dark, dull, and disagreeable. This may have been because he saw so little of it. Lectures and hospital attendance were confining; although he sometimes attended Friends meetings he seldom made even a short excursion into the country, and during a year's residence in London he never once traveled more than twenty miles from the city.[11] Despite this, however, London had its effect upon him, changing him from the plain and pacifist Quaker he had been when he came abroad in the summer of 1775. He became increasingly concerned with

[9] Hutchinson to Pemberton, April 7, 1776.
[10] Hutchinson to Pemberton, 6 mo. 12, 1776.
[11] Hutchinson to Catherine Milnor (his mother), December 20, 1775, and June 24, 1776; Hutchinson to Mary Pemberton, June 13–July 26, 1776.

reports of public affairs at home, and English friends stimulated his concern by constantly asking him for news and opinions. Though careful not to offend his uncle by discussing politics, he could hardly conceal where his loyalty lay. "I have too great an affection for my Country not to feel its distresses," he wrote; "its dearness to me causes me to share in the troubles, partake of the Calamities, and sympathise with the afflictions that now surround it. It is my constant wish & prayer that a reconciliation may take place, but it should be a constitutional one; any other would be only trifling, and give rise to future disputes. Oh! that the voice of Justice and reason could but be heard. They would have a much better effect than the mouth of the Cannon, or the Point of the Bayonet."[12] Israel Pemberton's careful scheme to shield his protégé from the passions and divisions of war had had but scant success.

Traveling from England to America in the summer of 1776 was, as Hutchinson quickly learned, no easy matter for a civilian. The packets were discontinued, and every merchant vessel risked capture. Some medical students, desperate to return, actually joined the British army as surgeons, intending to desert as soon as they reached America. Hutchinson rejected that alternative but he weighed others anxiously, for each week's delay added to his expenses, which were already greater, he feared, than Pemberton had bargained for. Then he heard that he might find passage from France. Dr. Fothergill advised him to try, and, as Hutchinson departed, gave the young man a final admonition about his future: "There is no doubt of thy getting into immediate employment—but alas the [Pennsylvania] Hospital—I wish it may not be in other hands—at least be filled with the wounded and distressed. This is one reason that makes me urgent for thy return. Most probably the Post of Surgeon to a Regiment may be offerd, if it can be decently declined it would be best, notwithstanding the present advantages—It would be out of character. In the Hospital thy services would be great, and thy progress tho more slow would be more certain...." Fothergill wrote a recommendation to Pemberton that was similar in substance.[13]

At Nantes Hutchinson found the *Sally*, Captain Rollins, bound for Philadelphia with military stores for the rebels. There, too, just before the *Sally*

[12] Hutchinson to Pemberton, 12 mo. 20, 1775.
[13] Fothergill to Hutchinson, 9 mo. 9, 1776; Fothergill to Pemberton, 10 mo. 5, 1776; Hutchinson to Catherine Milnor, September 20, 1776; Crafton & Colson to Alexander Delporte, October 12, 1776; Hutchinson to Pemberton, 6 mo. 12, 1776.

sailed, Hutchinson met Dr. Franklin, who had left America on October 26 and was resting a few days before proceeding to Paris to begin his work as American agent to France. Franklin gave his fellow-townsman dispatches for Congress, which the latter assured Franklin he would deliver or, should the *Sally* "be so unfortunate as to fall into the hands of any of the Piratical Cruisers of Britain," sink.[14]

The westward voyage was long, stormy, and uncomfortable; only the company of Dr. Hugh Williamson, another American physician, made it tolerable. The captain was frequently ill, the first mate was incompetent, and food ran low. Relief came a few days off the Delaware Capes, when the *Sally* encountered the American vessel *Wasp*. That day they dined on fresh pork, turnips, meat tongue, and potatoes, with plum pudding and claret. Mindful of the dispatches he carried, Hutchinson transferred to the *Wasp*, as did Williamson, but they had to leave most of their baggage behind. Put ashore in a strong surf a few miles south of Indian River, the travelers made their way to Lewes, where Rev. Dr. Matthew Wilson put them up and gave them a full account of events in America since Franklin's departure in October. Late at night on March 16 Hutchinson reached Philadelphia, where he delivered his letters to Robert Morris and learned that the *Sally* had been taken by the enemy.[15]

His homecoming was not entirely cheerful. He had a cold, caught when the surf drenched him as he came ashore. He had lost his clothes, surgical instruments, the medical notes and manuscripts written during a year in London, and many books, magazines, and political pamphlets. He had also lost two boxes of medicines, badly needed in the United States, which he had intended to use when setting up practice or to sell to defray the costs of his studies. On top of all this, he knew that by carrying political dispatches he

---

[14] Hutchinson to Franklin, "Thursday," Franklin MSS, 40: 165, American Philosophical Society Library.

[15] Hutchinson, Journal, February 25–March 16, 1777; *Pennsylvania Gazette*, March 19, 1777. This issue of the *Gazette* contained what may be Hutchinson's earliest political contribution to the newspapers. One of the passengers on the *Sally*—it could have been only Hutchinson or Williamson—was quoted as saying that the Declaration of Independence had "not in the least altered the sentiments of our friends in England, nor diminished their number. Those who are the real friends of liberty, now openly avow that the Americans are justifiable in their revolt from Great Britain . . . [and are] firmly persuaded that should the Americans be reduced to a state of slavery, their own liberty, or even the semblance of it, could not long survive."

had been guilty of an unneutral, unquakerly act of which his uncle, to whom he owed so much, could not approve.

Though Pemberton was hardly pleased with his nephew's political opinions and conduct and could do little to overcome the bad impression they made on Philadelphia Friends, among whom Hutchinson might have expected to build his practice, he gave the young man what help he could. He at once sent inquiries to New York about the captured trunks, requesting his correspondents to exert themselves to find and reclaim them, especially the sixteen volumes of notes of medical lectures. The return of such articles would not have been unprecedented in eighteenth-century warfare, but apparently Hutchinson's baggage was not recovered.[16] Pemberton showed further interest in his nephew when he supported his appointment as a physician to the Pennsylvania Hospital on May 12. Hutchinson was only twenty-five, the youngest physician yet named to the staff. Thus Hutchinson and Pemberton followed Dr. Fothergill's advice, that it would be better for the young surgeon to serve on the Hospital staff than to accept a commission in the army.

But a berth in the Pennsylvania Hospital was no haven from war's alarms and convulsions. Even Quaker neutrals were no longer safe. In September, on orders of the Pennsylvania Committee of Safety, Pemberton was seized, jailed, and carried off to imprisonment with other suspected persons. Hutchinson exerted himself in every way he could to represent his uncle's interests, by watching his property, writing him almost daily about events in Philadelphia, supporting a suit for a writ of habeas corpus, even by following him to Reading, where the prisoners stayed a short time; but all was without success. Pemberton was confined at Winchester, Virginia, for eight months in the fall and winter of 1777–78.[17] Meanwhile, Hutchinson had offered his services to care for the wounded of the battle of Germantown on October 4, and on December 1, 1777, he accepted appointment as Senior Surgeon of the Flying Hospital of the Middle Department and joined the American Army at Valley Forge.[18] By this act he broke from his Quaker heritage and relations.

[16] Pemberton to William McAdam, 3 mo. 24, 1777 (draft); Pemberton to Andrew Eliot, 3 mo. 25, 1777 (draft).

[17] Pemberton to Hutchinson, September 15 and thereafter to November 7, 1777; Robert Morton, "Diary . . . 1777," *Pennsylvania Magazine of History and Biography*, 1 (1877): 2, 9–10, 37 (hereafter cited as *Pa. Mag. Hist. Biog.*).

[18] Pemberton to Hutchinson, October 5, 1777; William Shippen, Jr., Appointment, December 1, 1777.

Little is known of his career in the army. About Valley Forge, where Charles Willson Peale painted his portrait, Hutchinson wrote afterwards that "there was such a want of Lancets that numbers of the regimental surgeons were without one, and that in June, 1778, when the army left Valley Forge, the sick in Camp amounted to near 3000." With one junior surgeon and a few regimental surgeons, Hutchinson was detailed to stay with them.[19] Because of his absence, he was not re-elected to the Pennsylvania Hospital staff in 1778, but on July 31 he was named (with Benjamin Rush) inspector of sickly vessels and was appointed surgeon of the Pennsylvania State Navy. The duties of the latter post were not burdensome, for the State Navy was neither large nor active; that summer Hutchinson went as a volunteer on General John Sullivan's expedition against Rhode Island. He returned in the fall, made a report on the medical requirements of the Navy, and on February 18, 1779, capped his un-Friendly behavior in war by marrying out of meeting. The bride was Lydia Biddle, daughter of John Biddle and sister of Colonel Owen Biddle, a lapsed Quaker. For martial and marital offenses against the Quaker discipline, Hutchinson was disowned on February 26, 1779.[20] In the ensuing years he received other appointments of a quasi-military kind— director-general and physician-in-chief of the state militia in 1780, director of hospitals, and physician and surgeon-general of the Commonwealth.[21]

Military service, however, was much less to Hutchinson's taste than politics; in the political upheavals that followed the Declaration of Independence and the creation of the Pennsylvania state government in 1776 he found an additional career. A man of heroic girth, friendly and affable, he got along well with everyone; his clear mind and trenchant writing style made him a useful ally in wars of the partisan press; and he was almost entirely without personal political ambitions. For a few months in 1780 he served as a member

[19] *Pa. Mag. Hist. Biog.*, 39 (1915): 221; Charles C. Sellers, *Portraits by Charles Willson Peale*, in *Trans. Amer. Philos. Soc.*, 42, pt. 1 (1952): 108.

[20] Marriage certificate, February 18, 1779; William Wade Hinshaw, *Encyclopedia of American Quaker Genealogy* (Ann Arbor, Mich., 1936), 2: 561. By this marriage Hutchinson became a brother-in-law of General James Wilkinson, who corresponded with him on personal and political matters; see *Pa. Mag. Hist. Biog.*, 12 (1888): 55–64, and 56 (1932): 33–55.

[21] Hutchinson, "Return of the sick belonging to the Pennsylvania State Navy," December 6, 1778, Gratz Collection, American Physicians, Historical Society of Pennsylvania; *Colonial Records of Pennsylvania*, 11: 543, 641; 12: 267, 323, 445; 13: 76; 14: 71; 15: 356, 640; 16: 82; *Pa. Archives*, 1st ser., 7: 408; 8: 496–97; 10: 178; 6th ser., 3: 968.

of the Assembly; it was the only public office he ever held, and he was defeated in the election for a full term.[22] In state politics he was a Radical, that is, a supporter of the Constitution of 1776. The causes and slogans that won his allegiance were like those that his father, in other circumstances, had supported thirty years before. From the close of the Revolution onward he achieved increasing influence in political councils, and he acquired quite a popular reputation as a partisan. In 1784 a satirist described him as follows:[23]

> See how the Dr. waddles through the throng,
> With Falstaff's belly, Liliputian's tongue,
> A beef-head bully—some has said a calf,—
> And that a goose has got more brains by half—
> That may be true—and further of this nibbler
> Some folks have said that he's a party scribbler!

Yet he was never doctrinaire, irresponsible, or inhumane. When a Bucks County cousin was seized on suspicion of trading with the enemy, Hutchinson quietly procured his release the next day. Moved by the sufferings of American civilians driven from their homes when the British army occupied Charleston, he served on a committee authorized by Congress to raise a fund for their relief. On an occasion when Philadelphia Radicals talked angrily of seizing the wives and children of absent Tories and sending them into the British lines in New York, Hutchinson was one of the moderates who opposed the scheme and deflected the ill-advised patriotic zeal.[24] He showed a similar sensible attitude in the reorganization of the Medical Department of the College of Philadelphia in 1779.

In that year the Pennsylvania Assembly removed the trustees of the College of Philadelphia on a charge of Loyalist sympathies, vested the property in a new board composed of officers of state and some other persons of Radical politics, and called the new institution the University of the State of Pennsylvania. Hutchinson was one of the new trustees. He was appointed at once

[22] *Pa. Archives*, 6th ser., 11: 350.

[23] *The Philadelphiad* (Philadelphia, 1784), 1: 50. The Tory poet Joseph Stansbury had described Hutchinson in similar terms: "that great bull calf—a gander has more brains by half"; Winthrop Sargent, *The Loyal Verse of Joseph Stansbury and Doctor Jonathan Odell* (Albany, 1860), p. 43.

[24] Robert L. Brunhouse, *The Counter-Revolution in Pennsylvania, 1776–1790* (Harrisburg, 1942), pp. 74–75; Samuel R. Fisher, "Journal," *Pa. Mag. Hist. Biog.*, 41 (1917): 297; William Bingham and others to ——, July 31, 1781 (circular), Gratz Collection, American Physicians, Historical Society of Pennsylvania; Worthington C. Ford *et al.*, eds., *Journals of the Continental Congress, 1774–1789*, 21: 786.

with Dr. Thomas Bond and Dr. William Shippen, Sr., to propose a plan to revive the medical school and re-establish it "on the most respectable footing." This was no easy task in 1780, for, in addition to political dissensions within the state, the former medical professors, who had not often or long been on amicable terms before, were now deeply divided by the bitter quarrel over the conduct of Dr. John Morgan and Dr. William Shippen, Jr., as successive heads of the Army's medical services. Morgan and Benjamin Rush refused to serve on the faculty with Shippen, while Shippen and his friends, both in and out of the profession, did nothing to let the feud die. To fill the empty posts the trustees elected Hutchinson professor of practice on July 2, 1781, but he declined. On November 7 they elected him professor of chemistry; but, though students looked forward to his lectures, on September 10, 1783, he declined that appointment too.

In 1789, when the Conservatives had been returned to power in Pennsylvania, the surviving trustees of the College of Philadelphia were restored. There were now two colleges in the city—the College of Philadelphia and the University of the State of Pennsylvania, and each had a medical school. Hutchinson accepted election as professor of chemistry and materia medica in the University on December 19, 1789. A union of the two institutions was obviously the only reasonable course. Hutchinson was a member of the committee on union, which was accomplished in 1791; having resigned his trusteeship, he was elected professor of chemistry in the new University of Pennsylvania on January 23, 1792.[25]

In the decade after the return of peace Hutchinson, now in his early thirties, began to take part in a variety of local activities. He was elected a member of the American Philosophical Society on April 16, 1779, and in 1782 was elected corresponding secretary; he served thereafter on several committees whose proposals led to the revival of the Society by procuring a charter and erecting a hall (to which he contributed £5). He was a member of the committee which solicited funds for André Michaux, until it was discovered that that Frenchman's plans for a botanizing tour of America had political purposes. Hutchinson had indicated on joining the Society that he had special interests in natural history and chemistry and in medicine and anatomy, but he appears to have taken little part in the Society's scientific

[25] University of Pennsylvania, Trustee's Minutes, December 9, 1779, *et passim*; Joseph Carson, *History of the Medical Department of the University of Pennsylvania* (Philadelphia, 1869), pp. 89–91.

work. He wrote no papers, although occasionally he was appointed to judge others'.[26] He presented a collection of shells from the Rappahannock River in Virginia to Pierre E. DuSimitière's museum in 1779, and in 1784 was one of the solicitors of subscriptions for the construction of an air balloon;[27] but these actions, like those within the Society, indicate no more than a mild interest in science.

Hutchinson's career in the College of Physicians was similar. He was one of the founders, served for the first two years as secretary, and at the time of his death was in his second term as a censor. He was on one committee to prepare a pharmacopoeia and on another to seek a charter from the legislature.[28] Otherwise he appears not to have played an active role or to have had discernible influence. Despite his undergraduate promise in chemistry and his almost unrivaled training and experience in surgery, he appears never to have written a word on either subject.

Hutchinson was one of the original incorporators of the Philadelphia Medical Society in 1792, a contributor to the Philadelphia Dispensary, and an inspector of the Humane Society. He was a member of the Pennsylvania Society for Promoting the Abolition of Slavery, and also of the first Society of Visitors of Peale's Museum in 1792. This last appointment may have been made in recognition of his professional standing; probably it owed as much to the fact that he was Peale's family doctor and that he and Peale were political cronies of long standing.[29]

Meanwhile, Mrs. Hutchinson had died, leaving the doctor with a young son to care for. On November 13, 1786, he married his second wife, Sydney, daughter of Joseph and Sydney (Evans) Howell, "a sweet looking young woman" some years younger than himself. One acquaintance called their entertainment "superb," and they had General Washington to dinner at least once during the Federal Convention summer. Sydney Hutchinson bore the doctor two sons, Israel Pemberton and Randall, and a daughter. Young James, the son by Hutchinson's first wife, received his M.D. from the University of Pennsylvania in 1803. I. Pemberton Hutchinson, after serving some time as a United States consul in Portugal, returned to Philadelphia, where

[26] Henry Phillips, "Early Proceedings of the American Philosophical Society," *Proc. Amer. Philos. Soc.*, 22 (1884–85): 102 *et seqq.*

[27] Pierre E. DuSimitière, Memoranda, 1774–83, Library of Congress; *Pennsylvania Gazette*, June 30, 1784.

[28] College of Physicians, Minutes, June 3, 1788, *et seqq.*

[29] Charles C. Sellers, *Charles Willson Peale* (Philadelphia, 1947), 2: 46.

the city directories listed him as "gent." Randall was admitted to the bar and later held appointments as clerk of the Mayor's Court and prothonotary. But Hutchinson saw no part of his sons' careers, not even their beginnings. As for his daughter, Catherine, he died the day she was born, and she died two months later.[30]

Throughout these years, of course, Hutchinson carried on his practice. It was almost his only source of income. As a physician at the Pennsylvania Hospital, to whose staff he was reappointed in November, 1779, he used his personal and political influence to increase the institution's funds. Professionally he took the surgical and obstetrical cases as his specialty—he delivered the child of Mary Girard, the merchant's crazy wife—but, like all the staff, looked after the sick as well. Samuel Coates, one of the Hospital managers, recorded in his journal the amusing story of how one of the insane patients enticed the doctor into her cell, locked him in, and then escaped. Hutchinson's cries at last brought someone to release him, and Polly was eventually found and brought back, "in high Glee . . . Exulting in the trick she had played upon the doctor."[31] In addition, Hutchinson's appointments as inspector of sickly vessels and physician of the state military and naval forces were periodically renewed, sometimes under different titles; he held the former until his death in 1793.

With the adoption of the Federal Constitution in 1788 and the final defeat of the Radicals in Pennsylvania in the following year, Hutchinson's political activity came to a brief halt. However, new issues on both state and national levels soon developed or were created; parties appeared, or reappeared under new names; and Hutchinson, aligning himself with the anti-Federalists, the Jeffersonians, and the friends of France in national politics (as he had been on the Radical side in state affairs), found fresh release for his talents.

In the state gubernatorial election of 1790 he played only a modest role, for Thomas Mifflin, whom he supported, was overwhelmingly the popular choice. The congressional election of 1792, however, was a lively contest, and Hutchinson was especially active. With Alexander James Dallas and

[30] Marriage certificate, November 13, 1786; Ann Warder, "Diary," *Pa. Mag. Hist. Biog.*, 18 (1894): 56–57; John C. Fitzpatrick, ed., *Diaries of George Washington* (Boston, 1925), 3: 235.
[31] Francis R. Packard, *History of Medicine in the United States* (New York, 1931), 1: 210; Morton and Woodbury, *Pennsylvania Hospital*, p. 138; Pennsylvania Hospital, Managers' Minutes, November 9, December 12, 1779.

Jonathan Dickinson Sergeant, he was among the principal Democratic managers who drew up the slate and then sold it to the party as a "Rights of Man ticket." Throughout the spring and summer Hutchinson carried on confidential political correspondence with Democrats in western Pennsylvania, wrote squibs and letters for the Democratic press, and, keeping himself alert to Federalist moves, thwarted some of the opposition's designs.[32] Though the Federalist cause probably suffered little as a result of Hutchinson's exertions, that of the Republicans steadily improved. The vehemence and bitterness of his opponents' remarks are a measure of his success and influence. Senator William Maclay was discussing the defense of the frontier with Albert Gallatin and several other westerners one night when

Dr. Hutchinson came in, greasy as a skin of oil and puffing like a porpoise. . . . He had a pretty tale to tattle over, quite new, quite *à la* Doctor, quite medical. Is the town sickly, Doctor? No, no; yes, yes, for the season. Accident, accident; half a family struck down yesterday. They had fed on pheasant. All who had eaten affected; all the doctors called; discharged the offensive food; recovered; the craws of the pheasants examined; laurel leaves found in them. The death of Judge Bryan explained; he and his wife ate pheasant; both felt torpid; she evacuated, he died. And thus we were entertained with the belchings of this bag of blubber for half an hour. I took my hat and left them.[33]

Hutchinson and his fellow-Jeffersonians were given a fresh symbol and focus for their ambitions and discontents in the spring of 1793. A new French minister, Edmond Genet, came to the United States to solicit American aid for France in its war with Europe. From Charleston, where he landed, Citizen Genet moved slowly toward Philadelphia, making undiplomatic speeches everywhere, encouraging inflammatory editorials and resolutions, creating emotional pressures that he imagined would force Washington's administration into open support of the French government. In Philadelphia, the ultimate focal point of these pressures, Hutchinson helped organize the public meeting at which an address of congratulation was delivered to Genet; and, with David Rittenhouse and others, he founded a Democratic Society to sustain and channel the enthusiasm Genet had created and to turn it to advantage in domestic politics. As it turned out, Genet overreached

[32] Harry M. Tinkcom, *The Republicans and Federalists in Pennsylvania, 1790–1801* (Harrisburg, 1950), pp. 35–40, 53–68; *Pa. Mag. Hist. Biog.*, 12 (1888): 372–73; Nathaniel Irwin to Hutchinson, October 3, 1792, and James Hanna to Hutchinson, October 16, 1792, Society Collection, Historical Society of Pennsylvania.
[33] Edgar S. Maclay, ed., *Journal of William Maclay* (New York, 1890), pp. 390–91.

himself, Washington was not intimidated, moderate-minded men prevailed, and the Frenchman's mission failed.

The political passions that Hutchinson and the Democratic Society had aroused remained high throughout mid-summer; and their support increased. Charles Caldwell, a recent graduate of the University of Pennsylvania in medicine, was one who applied for membership.[34] Then in August a new storm broke over Philadelphia which completely overwhelmed Genet, the Democratic Society, even any thought of France, kings, and revolution. A malignant fever appeared in Water Street.

By mid-August the number of deaths was increasing at an alarming rate, and rumors were multiplying and spreading rapidly through the city, terrifying the citizens. In these circumstances, on August 21 Governor Mifflin asked Hutchinson, as inspector of sickly vessels, to make an inquiry. The doctor did so, walking through the infected parts of the city, and on August 24 asked the physicians in town for their opinions. Dr. Rush, who had been saying privately that the disease was imported and who had called it yellow fever, now qualified both opinions: "Whether propagated . . . by contagion, or produced by the original exhalation from the Wharf, I cannot tell. It puts on all the intermediate forms between a mild Remittent, and the worst degree of typhus gravior," he wrote; "I have not seen a fever of so much Malignity, so general, since the year 1762." Hutchinson on August 27 transmitted the doctors' views to the health officer of the city, with his own conclusion that the disease had not been imported.[35] Accordingly, no quarantine was established in the port.

Meanwhile, Mayor Clarkson of Philadelphia had turned to the College of Physicians for advice. In a special meeting on Sunday, August 25, which Hutchinson attended, the physicians discussed the epidemic and the most promising methods of combating it. Hutchinson was put on a committee to draft directions for the public. The report was approved by the College on August 26 and was published the next day. The doctors warned against fatigue and unnecessary intercourse with the sick, prescribed clean, airy rooms, directed that the houses of the sick should be marked and that the

[34] Caldwell to Hutchinson, August 1, 1793.

[35] Benjamin Rush, *An Account of the Bilious Remitting Yellow Fever as it appeared in the City of Philadelphia, in the Year 1793* (Philadelphia, 1794), pp. 15–26. (The original of Rush's letter to Hutchinson is in the Hutchinson Papers.) See also John H. Powell, *Bring Out Your Dead* (Philadelphia, 1949), *passim*; Packard, *History of Medicine*, 2: 121–22; College of Physicians, Minutes, August 25, 26, 1793.

tolling of funeral bells should stop, and, among other things, suggested that a public hospital be established. There was now no doubt that yellow fever had spread through a large part of the waterfront area. Those who read the directions closely might also suspect that the doctors did not know what to do about it.

Though Dr. Hutchinson may have been uncertain where the fever came from, he knew that it was serious and would be fatal to many. Charles Biddle relates how the doctor urged him to take Mrs. Biddle out of town: in her presence Hutchinson would say only that the Biddles ought to leave. To Biddle, however, as they stood at the door, he confided that he had never seen anything that alarmed him so much, but that as a physician he felt that it was his duty to remain; taking Biddle's hand, he bade him farewell, saying it was unlikely they should meet again. And then he turned back.[36] The few glimpses recorded of Hutchinson in the next few days are of a man of humanity and quiet courage. Elizabeth Drinker heard that he had personally put a fever victim into a coffin, when no one else would do it. Biddle was told how the doctor, visiting a poor old woman, found her in a small closed room which stank almost unbearably; he opened the windows and sat with her for a while.[37]

On the evening of August 30 Hutchinson dined with Thomas Jefferson at the latter's place at Gray's Ferry. They must have talked of politics, especially of Genet's visit, the prospects of the Democratic-Republican Party, and the role of the Democratic Clubs; they certainly talked about the fever. That night Hutchinson fell ill. Dr. Adam Kuhn treated him, and, after Kuhn came down with the fever, William Currie and Benjamin Smith Barton cared for him. Rush, who was convinced that heavy bleeding and purging were the only proper treatment, urged them upon his colleague; but Hutchinson refused them. For a week his condition varied; sometimes he felt well enough to get out of bed, walk about the house, and even do some work; but on September 6 he died.[38]

[36] Charles Biddle, *Autobiography* (Philadelphia, 1883), pp. 255–56.
[37] Elizabeth Drinker, *Journal* (Philadelphia, 1889), p. 194; Biddle, *Autobiography*, pp. 255–56.
[38] L. H. Butterfield, ed., *Letters of Benjamin Rush*, 2: 648, 650, 651, 653, 675; W. S. W. Ruschenberger, *An Account of The Institution and Progress of the College of Physicians of Philadelphia* (Philadelphia, 1887), pp. 62–65. One of Hutchinson's apprentices also died; Matthew Carey, *A Short History of the Plague, or Malignant Fever lately prevalent in Philadelphia* . . . (Philadelphia, 1794), p. 88.

The death of such a well-known person increased the public's alarm. If the doctors could not save one of their own, what hope, people murmured, was there for ordinary folk? Moreover, Hutchinson's death became a sort of *cause célèbre* in the profession in Philadelphia. Rush, who had not been allowed in the sick room and had never seen Hutchinson, attacked Kuhn's mild prescriptions and vigorously asserted that his own treatment would have been successful. Kuhn, who had lost the patient, reported the case in full detail in lectures at the Medical School, sometimes hinting that, since Hutchinson had not recovered, his prescriptions must have been changed after he had to leave the case.[39]

As expected, politicians were also divided about Hutchinson's death. Gallatin, who had worked with him closely in Pennsylvania politics, sincerely mourned the loss of an adviser whose principles, integrity, and warmth of friendship "had attached me to him more than to any man in Philadelphia." Jefferson told James Madison that it was hard to know "whether the republican interest has suffered more by his death or Genet's extravagance." *Dunlap's American Daily Advertiser*, though allowing that Hutchinson might have gone to an extreme in support of the French Revolution, paid tribute to one it called a uniform friend of the people, who was animated by "the purest love of human nature and of human rights."[40]

No Federalist, of course, could agree with Dunlap's estimate or believe with Jefferson that the republic had suffered any loss by Hutchinson's death. Years afterward, reviewing the history of the republic with his old friend Jefferson, John Adams recalled, with characteristic exaggeration, that in the summer of 1793 a mob of 10,000 had been ready to drag Washington from the President's house into the streets and to force the government to abandon neutrality and declare war in favor of France. "The coolest and firmest Minds, even among the Quakers in Philadelphia," Adams continued, "have given their Opinion to me, that nothing but the Yellow Fever, which removed Dr. Hutchinson . . . from this World, could have saved the United States from a total Revolution of Government."[41]

[39] Ruschenberger, *College of Physicians*, pp. 62–65.
[40] Henry Adams, *Life of Albert Gallatin* (New York, 1879), p. 105; Paul L. Ford, ed., *The Writings of Thomas Jefferson* (New York, 1892–99), 6: 419; *Dunlap's American Daily Advertiser*, September 13, 1793.
[41] Adams to Jefferson, June 30, 1813, in *The Adams-Jefferson Letters*, ed. Lester J. Cappon (Chapel Hill, N.C., 1959), 2: 347.

James Hutchinson was in mid-career when he died; because his death was only one of thousands of premature deaths in Philadelphia in 1793, the loss could not easily be measured. Had he lived, continuing to perform much of the surgery at the Pennsylvania Hospital, Hutchinson might have been recognized as the ablest, as he was surely the best-trained, surgeon in the city before Philip Syng Physick established himself. In politics he probably would have become an increasingly powerful figure in the emerging party of Jefferson and, though he had shown little taste for public office, he might have been elected to the United States Senate, as Dr. George Logan was a few years later. He might, in short, have entered into the pantheon of heroes of the new republic, to be recalled by subsequent generations, in the words of Charles Biddle, as "a very able physician, and one of the best of men."[42]

[42] Pennsylvania Hospital, Managers' Minutes, 11 mo. 25, 1793.

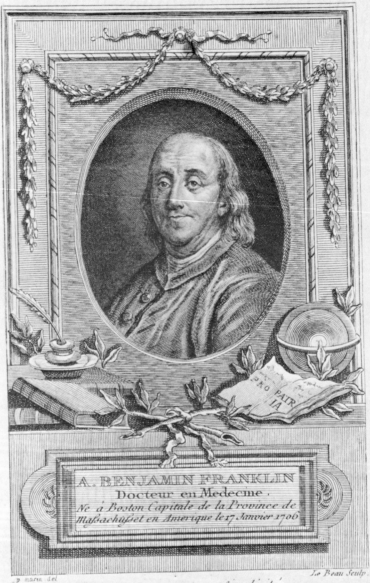

p maria del   le Beau Sculp.

A. BENJAMIN FRANKLIN

Docteur en Medecine,

Né à Boston Capitale de la Province de
Massachusset en Amerique le 17 Janvier 1706

Sa Vertu son Courage et sa Simplicité
De Sparte ont retracé le Caractere Antique
Et cher a la raison, cher à l'Humanité
Il Eclaira l'Europe et sauva l'Amerique

Benjamin Franklin
and the Practice of Medicine

Medicine was a branch of knowledge with which almost every educated man in the eighteenth century had some acquaintance. Laymen discussed medical principles as they did eclipses, humming birds, and Greek forms of government. They bought, read, and annotated medical texts, treated illnesses in their own households, sometimes even attended anatomical lectures. It is not surprising that in such an atmosphere Benjamin Franklin too should have been interested in medical science, or that he should have made discerning comments on health and disease and even prescribed remedies for the sick.

In Franklin's case the general climate of the age was reinforced by his special scientific interest. Among the books and gadgets and electrical apparatus in his library, for example, a visitor in 1787 saw a "glass machine for exhibiting the circulation of the blood in the arteries and veins of the human body." Because physicians had had formal scientific training and were likely as well to be rationalists with warm humanitarian sympathies, Franklin found them congenial, and he was closely associated with a number of them in both his experimental work and in his public career. With Cadwallader Colden, a medical graduate of Edinburgh, he discussed anatomical and physiological concepts; to Dr. Cadwalader Evans he explained his understanding of lead-poisoning; while Dr. Thomas Bond, his fellow-member of the Junto, was his fellow-founder of the Pennsylvania Hospital. European physicians were equally distinguished among Franklin's friends: the Quaker John Fothergill, friend of Pennsylvania's Holy Experiment, Franklin's personal physician in London, with whom he made a final effort to maintain peace between England and the colonies in the winter of 1775; Sir John Pringle, president of the Royal Society, who accompanied him on a tour of Holland and Germany; the French physician and physicist Dubourg, who published the first general edition of Franklin's writings. Physicians sent him prescriptions to test and assess; medical societies in London, Paris, and Edinburgh saw nothing incongruous in electing this philosopher to membership; and a French artist, engraving a portrait of Franklin, mistakenly but understandably characterized him as "docteur en médecine" [cf. portrait on cover]. Moreover, Franklin encouraged and guided a whole generation of American students abroad, from William Shippen and John Morgan to George Logan and Benjamin Waterhouse. Benjamin Rush, Caspar Wistar and Jonathan Elmer dedicated their inaugural dissertations to him.

Throughout his life Franklin was a willing publicist of medical information. He had definite theories of disease and therapy and, as was the case when he believed his ideas would benefit men, he urged them strongly and constantly in his publications and in private letters. He reprinted John Tennent's *Every Man His Own Physician,* recommending it to the public but warning that as Pennsylvania ipecac was stronger than the Virginia variety, the prescribed dosages should be modified accordingly. Franklin spread abroad other men's medical ideas as well. No sooner had he returned to England from a visit to Paris, for example, than he sent his friend Dubourg a copy of Thomas Dimsdale on smallpox inoculation which they had been discussing; and his parting gift to the Royal Society of Medicine in Paris was a copy of Haygarth on smallpox.

Smallpox was something about which he was deeply concerned through more than sixty years. It was a great killer, terrible and swift; as a result laymen as well as physicians devoted a good deal of thought and energy to measures of prevention and treatment. Franklin was an early advocate of inoculation, and never wavered in his support of it. His brother James' newspaper, the *New-England Courant,* it is true, had attacked inoculation, but that was because Cotton Mather endorsed it; and the Franklins were anti-clerical. In Philadelphia, where such rivalries did not prevail, the younger Franklin supported the new preventive measures and at every opportunity spread knowledge of improved methods of preparing the patient and administering the disease. In his newspaper, for example, he hailed the successful inoculation of Joseph Growdon during the Philadelphia epidemic of 1730-31 as proof of inoculation's relative safety; and in the moment of his greatest personal loss he took the occasion to reaffirm his complete confidence in the measure:

> Understanding 'tis a current Report, that my Son Francis, who died lately of the Small Pox, had it by Inoculation; and being desired to satisfy the Publick in that Particular, inasmuch as some People are, by that Report (join'd with others of the like kind, and perhaps equally groundless) deter'd from having the Operation perform'd on their Children, I do hereby sincerely declare, that he was not inoculated, but receiv'd the Distemper in the common Way of Infection: And I suppose the Report could only arise from its being my known Opinion, that Inoculation was a safe and beneficial Practice; and from my having said among my Acquaintance, that I intended to have my Child inoculated, as soon as he should have recovered sufficient Strength from a Flux with which he had been long afflicted.

In smallpox, as in other fields, Franklin was receptive to new ideas, willing to give them a hearing. Adam Thomson, for example, a Scots physician in Maryland, perfected a regimen of mercury, antimony, and quinine for preparing patients for inoculation. He came to Philadelphia in 1748 to urge and practice his method. Inevitably older physicians offered opposition. To give the newcomer a better audience Franklin proposed that the Trustees of the Academy of Philadelphia allow Thomson to lecture in the Academy building. This permission was granted, and when Thomson was charged with presumptuously declaring he had lectured "before the Trustees of the Academy," as though they were his patrons, Franklin printed a note in his defense. (And then, because Franklin was a merchant-printer as well, he printed Dr. John Kearsley's attack on the Thomsonian method.)

Repeatedly as the years passed Franklin collected statistics from towns where smallpox was epidemic. All the figures showed that taking smallpox by inoculation was many times safer than to receiving "in the natural way;" and Franklin spread the figures and his conclusion as widely as he could in private letters to physicians and others. In 1759 he presented statistics from a recent Boston epidemic, with the arguments based on them, as a preface to Dr. William Heberden's *Some Account of the Success of Inoculation for the Small-Pox.* Skilful, humane, and successful, Heberden was convinced that inoculation was so safe and desirable that it might and should be practiced by intelligent laymen; his pamphlet presented plain instructions, expressed, at Franklin's suggestion, in simple language, to enable any person to perform the operation and conduct the patient through the disease and convalescence. Franklin sent 1500 copies to America for free distribution by physicians and leading citizens.

And still he kept looking for ways to provide universal protection against this most deadly scourge. He told William Vassall of Boston, for example, that there was no need to go to New York to be inoculated, "since, as has been try'd here with Success, a dry Scab or two will communicate the Distemper by Inoculation, as well as fresh Matter taken from a Pustule and kept warm till apply'd to the Incision, and such might be sent you per Post from hence, cork'd up tight in a small Phial." Thus might the Deputy Postmaster-General for North America serve the public health.

Franklin did not, of course, confine the dissemination of ideas on medicine and medical care to smallpox. He made other "incursions into medicine," to use the phrase of a French commentator on the subject in 1956. At the height of a diphtheria epidemic in Boston in 1743, for example, Franklin sent there a letter (published soon thereafter in the *American Magazine and Historical Chronicle*) suggesting that the disease was the same described by the French traveller Tournefort in his *Voyage to the Levant* some years before and that the same remedies the Greeks used on Iona might be effective in Massachusetts.

Franklin never tired of propagandizing his conviction that fresh air, exercise, and temperance are essential to prevent disease and preserve health. "Wouldst thou enjoy a long Life, a healthy Body, and a vigorous Mind?" *Poor Richard* asked in 1742; then "bring thy Appetite into Subjection to Reason." Here was Franklin's basic principle of healthful living. Though he did not always practice it, he never forgot it; and whenever illness overtook him, he resumed his rational regimen, putting more reliance on moderation in food and drink, fresh air and gentle exercise than on the doctors' powders and potions.

Such notions as these were novel in an age of two-bottle men, who thought the night air noxious. As a youth Franklin had come upon a copy of Thomas

Tryon's seventeenth century *Way to Health, Long Life and Happiness.* Convinced by Tryon's arguments, but partly, it must be admitted, for economy's sake, young Franklin had become a vegetarian; and, though he resumed meat-eating, he often returned to the vegetarian diet for brief periods for reasons of health. "In general," he wrote, "mankind, since the improvement of cooking, eats about twice as much as nature requires. Suppers are not bad, if we have not dined, but restless nights naturally follow hearty suppers after full dinners. . . . Nothing is more common in newspapers than instances of people who, after eating a hearty supper, are found dead abed in the morning."

Franklin believed in exercise as stoutly as in temperate diet, and for the same reason—that medical treatment was uncertain. Exercise, he advised his son, was "of the greatest importance to prevent diseases, since the cure of them by physic is so very precarious." He advocated swimming as "one of the most healthy and agreeable" exercises, and himself swam when he was 70 years old; recommended that people walk when they could not swim, and swing dumb-bells in their rooms when they could not walk—as he did daily at 82. His sister Jane, ever mindful of his example and advice, took her exercise walking in Boston, even though offered a chaise and when she was "so weak I make but a Poor figure in the Street." Franklin's long summer journeys were undertaken partly to promote his health, which suffered in England from close confinement to business; and when he had to forego such vacations, as he did in his later years because of his stone, his health deteriorated noticeably.

Franklin was the great advocate of fresh air. The lack of it, he pointed out to English physicians, was a cause of high mortality in the manufacturing towns. "Our Physicians," he wrote in 1773, "have begun to discover that fresh Air is good for People in the Small-Pox and other Fevers. I hope in time they will find out that it does no harm to People in Health;" and he derided English fears of fresh air. "Many London families go out once a day to take the air," he remarked; "three or four persons in a coach, one perhaps sick; these three go three or four miles, or as many turns in Hyde Park, with the glasses both up close, all breathing over again the same air they brought out of town with them in the coach with the least change possible, and render'd worse and worse every moment. And this they call *taking the Air.*" John Adams has left an amusing account of Franklin's fervid advocacy of fresh air. Travelling together to New York, the two men shared a small room at an inn at New Brunswick, N. J. The window was open when they entered the room; Adams shut it tight at once. "Oh," said Franklin, "don't shut the window; we shall be suffocated." Adams declared he was afraid of the night air. "The air within this chamber will soon be, and indeed is now, worse than that without doors," Franklin replied firmly. "Come, open the window and come to bed, and I will convince you. I believe you are not acquainted with my theory of colds." And with that Franklin threw up the window. Poor Adams leaped into bed, and the Doctor, Adams recorded, "then began a harangue upon air and cold, and respiration and perspiration," which soon put Adams to sleep and, he believed, put Franklin to sleep as well, for the last words Adams remembered hearing from his companion were pronounced in a faraway drone as though Franklin were already losing consciousness.

Franklin's advocacy of cold air baths was widely known in the eighteenth century, and perhaps as widely marvelled at. He thought them less a shock to the system than cold water. "I rise almost every morning," he wrote, "and sit in my chamber without any clothes whatever, half an hour or an hour, according to the season, whether reading or writing. This practice is not in the least painful, but, on the contrary, agreeable." After all, he told Dr. Rush, people do not *catch* cold from being cold or wet; but because of poor ventilation, too rich a diet, and too little exercise. One of the unwritten medical classics is Franklin's treatise on colds; only an outline of it—a very full outline, be it said—survives; but like the great work he contemplated on the "Art of Virtue," it was never finished. So famous, indeed, was Dr. Franklin's air bath that some hygienists believed it should have a local habitation as well as a name: at least a German magazine in 1798 published a picture of Franklin's *Luftbad:* an attractive Chinese pavilion suited to a quiet corner of a romantic garden.

Franklin got closer to medical practice than publicizing medical knowledge and opinions, whether his own or others'. He practiced medicine—at least he prescribed for and treated the sick, sometimes in consultation with physicians, but not infrequently alone. A sister developed a cancer of the breast. Such a condition was generally thought to be incurable, "yet we have here in town," young Franklin wrote from Philadelphia, "a kind of shell made of some wood, cut at a proper time, by some man of great skill (as they say) which has done wonders in that disease among us, being worn for some time on the breast;" and he promised to borrow this miraculous shell to send to Boston for his sister to wear. On an occasion when another sister complained of shortness of breath, Benjamin suggested her condition might be relieved by spreading honey instead of butter on her bread at breakfast. This pressing medical advice on relations, friends and neighbors old Mrs. Franklin thought officious meddling in the doctors' business; but her son assured her that, as he always consulted a physician for any disorder in his family, she should regard his prescriptions as only a mark of his good will; and he kept right on giving advice. A year or so later, Franklin's brother John asked advice in some urinary trouble, and Benjamin promptly replied suggesting first the use of lime-water and soap—the remedy proposed by Dr. Whytt of Edinburgh—and then a catheter, and he had a Philadelphia silversmith make a sample, which he sent brother John with directions for modifying it.

A young woman of Philadelphia was afflicted by some violent and mysterious disease; her doctor, Thomas Bond, could do nothing; hopefully he invited

Franklin to visit the patient; and Franklin was present when, after a singularly extreme attack, the girl had a bowel movement and evacuated part of a rather long worm. Her sister sent Franklin a full account of the case. Again, when Dr. Samuel Johnson of New York was unable to visit Philadelphia because of illness, Franklin was ready with advice: "Don't imagine yourself thoroughly cured," he warned, "and so omit the use of the bark too soon. Remember to take the preventing doses faithfully . . . a dose or two every day for two or three weeks after the fits have left you . . . would not be amiss. If you take the powder mixed quick in a tea-cup of milk, 'tis no way disagreeable, but looks and even tastes like chocolate." And at St. Andrews to receive an honorary degree, Franklin was taken to see an undergraduate who was seriously ill; and that young man, who became Earl of Buchan, ever afterwards gratefully testified that Franklin's prescription had saved his life.

But it was, as one might expect, as an electrician that Franklin played his most active and intimate role as a practitioner of medicine. He was the first electrician in the world; and electricity—"the pure physic of the skies"—was believed by many to be the most powerful, because the most nearly divine, of all medicines. Certainly it seemed at first to offer benefit in cases of nervous disorders. The press in the late 1740s and early 1750s was filled with accounts of spectacular cures: the blind saw, the deaf heard, paralytics walked home after submitting to shocks from the miraculous fluid. Franklin did not fail to note that most of these "cures" took place in remote Italian, German or Russian villages, and were unsubstantiated; and he considered that even in less backward places some persons were "too premature in publishing their imaginations and expectations for real experiments." But patients given up as incurable grasped at any hope; soon they began to appeal to Franklin. He could not refuse, nor did he.

One of his earliest patients was old James Logan, the outstanding public figure and scholar of Pennsylvania for half a century until his death in 1751. In the early thirties he had encouraged and supported the young printer of the *Pennsylvania Gazette;* later the two men had corresponded happily on bookish matters, and Franklin frequently visited at Stenton, where Logan was assembling the great library he meant to give to the city of Philadelphia. Now, old and paralyzed, he sought whatever help the electric jars and bottles of his younger friend might give him. Another whom Franklin tried to help was Governor Jonathan Belcher of New Jersey, a man of 70, afflicted with what he called "the Common Paralytick disorder," or palsy. Otherwise, he told Franklin, he was pretty free from pain and sickness and commonly drank half a bottle of old madeira a day, in addition to water and small beer. A cautious man, Governor Belcher first sent a friend to discuss electrification with the Philadelphia doctors and with Franklin; satisfied with their opinions, he determined to undergo treatment, eagerly and gratefully accepted Franklin's offer to perform the experiment himself. Unfortunately, as it fell out, Franklin could not leave Philadelphia, but he shipped the equipment to Burlington, with specific instructions how to use it. It was his practice, Franklin explained later, to place the patient in a chair on an electric stool and draw a number of large, strong sparks from all parts of the affected limb or side. Then he charged fully two six-gallon glass jars and sent the united shock through the affected part. He repeated this three times a day.

Happily Belcher, who had now gone to Elizabeth, N. J., was able to call on his friend, the Reverend Aaron Burr, to operate Franklin's equipment. It is a moving scene—the old governor, bravely, hopefully submitting to this strange therapy which came out of bottles and points and wires which were manipulated by the reverend president of the College of New Jersey. Despite his own courage and President Burr's skill, however, Belcher felt no improvement, even after several applications.

No account of Belcher's case ever reached the London medical journals; and, since he was careful to keep the matter private, it is doubtful that any but his close friends and household knew about the treatment. But one of Franklin's cases, apparently a successful cure, was printed in a medical journal—the London *Medical Observations and Inquiries*—in 1757. It was reported by Cadwalader Evans, then a medical student in Philadelphia. C. B., aged 14,

> was seized with convulsion fits, which succeeded each other so fast, that she had near 40 in 24 hours after the first attack. She struggled with such violence in the fits, that three strong people could scarcely keep her in bed; after bleeding, blisters, with the use of anodynes and nervous medicines, they now abated in severity, and did not return above once or twice a day. It was thought to be occasioned by an obstruction of the *menses,* from imprudently exposing herself to cold, at the time of their appearance; therefore she was put on a course of gums, steel, bitters, &c. which succeeded in procuring that discharge in a pretty regular manner.
>
> Notwithstanding this, her disorder continued in one shape or other, or returned after an intermission of a month or two, at farthest. Sometimes she was tortured almost to madness with a cramp in different parts of the body; then with more general convulsions of the extremities, and a choaking deliquium; and, at times, with almost the whole train of hysteric symptoms.

These attacks continued for ten years, though the patient had good medical advice. At last, she determined to see what electricity could do for her, and in September 1752 went to Philadelphia and applied to Franklin. "I received four shocks morning and evening," she reported; "they were what they call 200 strokes of the wheel, which fills an eight gallon bottle, and indeed they were very severe. On receiving the first shock, I felt the fit very strong, but the second effectually carried it off; and thus it was every time I went through the operation; yet the symptoms gradually decreased, till at length they entirely left me." The patient continued in Philadelphia two weeks, and when she returned home Franklin gave her a bottle with which he instructed her to electrify herself every day for three weeks. Two years later she was still in good health.

Too often, of course, the results were negative, as Franklin knew they would be; and not all the improvements which patients made could properly be ascribed to the electrical treatment. To Sir John Pringle in 1757 Franklin summarized his experience in measured terms. He first observed "an immediately greater sensible Warmth in the lame Limbs that had receiv'd the Stroke;" the next morning the patients usually reported a pricking sensation in the paralyzed limbs during the night; and the limbs themselves seemed to have recovered strength and to be more capable of movement. Sometimes this improvement continued for five days, "but I do not remember that I ever saw any Amendment after the fifth Day." Seeing that improvement did not continue, the patients became restless and discouraged; most went home and relapsed; "so that I never knew any Advantage from Electricity in Palsies that was permanent. And how far the apparent temporary advantage might arise from the exercise in the patient's journey, and coming daily to my home, or from the spirits given by the hope of success, enabling them to exert more strength in moving their limbs, I will not pretend to say."

Yet confidence in the powers of electricity continued little abated, especially in rural areas and among quacks like the notorious James Graham, and even in London. Not long after Franklin reached England in 1757 Sir John Pringle begged him to electrise the epileptic daughter of the Duke of Ancaster; and a young Border squire, who had lost his hearing after an attack of smallpox, proposed coming to London to be electrised, if Franklin thought it would help. Similar expressions of confidence in electricity and Franklin greeted the old man when he reached France as an American agent in 1777. Some, who wanted his endorsement, claimed striking successes, like DeThourry of Caen, who told Franklin that of 60 patients treated electrically, only one had been harmed and only two or three had remained unaffected, all the rest—the qualification did not escape Franklin—"who persevered in treatment and whose malady was not of long standing, being cured or almost cured." Others asked only for information, and instruction, like Père Guinchard, a country priest who had bought an electrical machine to bring relief and cures to his beloved parishioners.

If faith in medical electricity was slow dying, it was partly because the philosophers kept observing new phenomena and unnoticed qualities which might have therapeutic value. Franklin's friend Dr. Jan Ingenhousz, physician to the Austrian Court, accidentally received a very severe shock. When he recovered, he told Franklin, he "felt the most lively joye in finding as I thought at the time, my judgment infinitely more acute. . . . What did formerly seem to me difficult to comprehend, was now become of an easy Solution. I found moreover a liveliness in my whole frame, which I never had observed before." This accident, together with two similar ones that had happened to Franklin, induced Ingenhousz to suggest to "the London mad-Doctors" that similar shocks should be administered to the insane at Bedlam, "thinking that, as I found myself my mental faculties improved and as the world well knows, that your mental faculties, if not improved by the two strokes you received, were certainly not hurt, by them, it might perhaps become a remedy to recover the mental faculties when lost. . . ." Ingenhousz had been unable to persuade either the "mad-Doctors" or anyone else to his view; but Franklin, as Ingenhousz asked, recommended electric shock treatment to the physician appointed by the British government to treat epileptic and insane persons.

Perhaps any discussion of Franklin and the practice of medicine should include some mention of him in the role of patient, sometimes John Fothergill's or Thomas Bond's, not seldom his own. Like so many of his contemporaries, he was often sick. From his personal letters one can compile a depressing catalogue of fevers, colds, bruises (he dislocated his shoulder in 1763 and had a severe fall when he was 82), eczema, gout and stone. Each of these he treated in his own way—usually by regulating his diet, by exercise and bathing; or, if he consulted the physicians, he followed their prescriptions only insofar as he thought them reasonable. Being Franklin's physician could have been no ordinary experience for a doctor. Whatever his "ails," he accepted them uncomplainingly: "when I consider how many terrible diseases the human body is liable to," he wrote philosophically when he was 82—and he repeated the sentiment many times, once within a few weeks of his death at 84—"I comfort myself that only three incurable ones have fallen to my share, viz. the gout, the stone, and old age; and that these have not yet deprived me of my natural cheerfulness, my delight in books and enjoyment of social conversation."

As a young man of 21 Franklin had a severe pleurisy that was almost fatal. Eight years later he had a second attack, which was so violent that his left lung suppurated. Thereafter, though his health was as good as anyone in the eighteenth century could reasonably expect, Franklin suffered often, and frequently severely, from colds, especially after middle age. His letters home from London contain many references to them. In September 1758 he wrote Deborah that he had had "a most violent Cold;" and 18 months later he was "much indispos'd with an Epidemical Cold" that had "lain greatly" in his head. Soon after reaching London again in 1764 he was "severely handled" for ten or twelve days "by a most violent Cold, that has worried me extremely;" and two months later he was still weak from it. Another year he had "the epidemical Cold that every body has had," and still again it was "a violent Cold" that so affected his head and eyesight that he could hardly write. An undated scrap of paper among Franklin's surviving manuscripts records the onset of one of his attacks:

Monday	—Din'd at Club—Beef
Tuesday	—at Mr. Foxcroft's—Fish

Wednesday   —Dolly's—Beefstake. Felt symptoms of
    Cold—Fullness

Thursday   —Mr. Walker's—Beef
    Predicted it.

Friday at home—Mutton
    little Soreness of Throat

Saturday   —Club—Veal

Sunday morng. —Had a good Night but U[rine] has deposited
    a reddish fine Sand.

More disagreeable and certainly more alarming to Franklin were the fits of dizziness that overtook him and sometimes lasted for as long as several weeks. He felt the symptoms on reaching England in 1757: giddiness, a humming noise in head, and now and then "little faint twinkling Lights. And my Head feels tender." These attacks may have arisen from excessive eating and insufficient exercise; though he had one such attack when he was supervising the construction of forts on the Pennsylvania frontier in 1756, and must have been eating simply and getting a good deal of physical exercise. All the same, bleeding and a moderated diet seemed to help, even when the dizziness was but one of a whole complex of symptoms. From Christmas till Easter, he wrote his wife in the spring of 1770, he had

> a disagreeable Giddiness hanging about me, which however did not hinder me from being about and doing Business. In the Easter Holidays being at a Friend's House in the Country, I was taken with a sore Throat, and came home half strangled. From Monday till Friday, I could swallow nothing but Barley Water and the like. I was bled largely, and purged two or three times. On Friday came on a Fit of the Gout, from which I had been free five Years. Immediately the inflammation and Swelling in my Throat disappeared; my Foot swelled greatly, and I was confined about three Weeks; since which I am perfectly well, the Giddiness and every other disagreeable Symptom having quite left me.

Franklin's gout, thanks to an amusing bagatelle he wrote about it, is probably his best known illness. He first felt its twinges in 1749, and thereafter to the end of his life he had it frequently, sometimes only an intimation of the pain, but often a severe attack that incapacitated him for several weeks. The treatment was the usual one of a plain diet; and Franklin himself discovered that the pain in his foot could sometimes be relieved by thrusting it out of the bedclothes and exposing it all night to the cold air. But Franklin was quite philosophical about the gout. The irritation and inconvenience it caused him were nothing compared to terrible afflictions he might have suffered. "People who live long," he told a sympathizing friend, "who will drink of the cup of life to the very bottom, must expect to meet with some of the usual dregs. . . ." He liked to think it was not a disease at all, but a remedy, since he always felt more vigorous physically and more alert mentally after an attack.

One such attack, Franklin believed, cured an eczema that had persisted for 14 years. Once it covered all his body except face and hands; he asked Sir John Pringle's advice; but nothing cured it and only warm bathing gave any relief. But in 1788, when it was "as bad as ever," the gout attacked again,

> without very much pain, but a swelling in both feet, which at last appeared also in both knees, and then in my hands. As these swellings increased and extended, the other malady diminished and at length disappeared entirely. Those swellings have now some time since begun to fall, and are now almost gone; perhaps the cutaneous disease may return, or perhaps it is worn out . . . I am on the whole much weaker than when it began to leave me. But possibly that may be the effect of age, for I am now near eighty-three, the age of commencing decrepitude.

If Franklin's gout is the disease posterity knows best, his stone was by all odds his most grievous affliction. It began to trouble him in 1779 when he was 73, and the symptoms became increasingly noticeable in the next few years. In 1782, after a very severe attack, he seriously considered an operation, but the surgeons who were consulted—John Hunter was one—advised against it because of his age, proposed control by diet, and urged the patient to hope for the best.

Thereafter Franklin ate more sparingly, drank no wine, avoided jolting carriages, and exercised only gently with dumbbells. By these means, the stone remained bearable for some time, and Franklin kept his wonted cheerfulness, read and wrote as usual, enjoyed company, slept well, and showed no slackening of his powers. "If I can prevent its growing larger," he told John Jay in 1784, "which I hope to do by abstemious living and gentle exercise, I can go on pretty comfortably with it to the end of my Journey, which can now be at no great distance."

Despite Franklin's regimen, the stone grew and his discomfort increased. By 1787 it caused him great pain to stand, walk or pass water, and he was reasonably comfortable only when he sat or lay abed. Friends and well-wishers pressed cures on him; he told the French naturalist Buffon, who sought advice in a similar condition, that he tried many of them, but without perceiving good effects from any, except, perhaps, blackberry jelly, which he took before retiring each night. Soon, however, the pain was so excruciating and so constant that he had to take laudanum, but the drug destroyed his appetite. In his last months he was "totally emaciated," little remaining of him, he told a friend, "but a Skeleton with a Skin."

During most of March 1790 Franklin was "quite free from pain;" not having to take laudanum, his appetite returned and he recovered some of his strength. But death was near; when it came it was as his old enemy pleurisy. His doctor John Jones described his last days:

> About sixteen days before his death, he was seized with a feverish disposition, without any particular symptoms attending it till the third or fourth day, when he complained of a pain in his left breast, which increased till it became extremely acute, attended by

a cough and laborious breathing. During this state, when the severity of his pains drew
forth a groan of complaint, he would observe, that he was afraid he did not bear them
as he ought; acknowledging his grateful sense of the many blessings he had received
from the Supreme Being, who had raised him, from small and low beginnings, to such
high rank and consideration among men; and made no doubt but that his present afflictions were kindly intended to wean him from a world in which he was no longer fit
to act the part assigned him. In this frame of body and mind, he continued until five
days before his death, when the pain and difficulty of breathing entirely left him, and
his family were flattering themselves with the hopes of his recovery; but an imposthume
which had formed in his lungs, suddenly burst, and discharged a quantity of matter,
which he continued to throw up while he had power; but, as that failed, the organs of
respiration became gradually oppressed; a calm, lethargic state succeeded; and on the
17th instant [April, 1790], about eleven o'clock at night, he quietly expired, closing a
long and useful life of eighty-four years and three months.

But, to return to Franklin and the practice of medicine. What there remains
to say—or to say again—is that in all Franklin did both as a publicist and a
practitioner of medicine he revealed the inquiring intelligence and easy competence which distinguish every facet of his many-sided genius. He thought
clearly and constructively about health and disease, developed some sound theories
and proposed sensible practices, and was ever mindful who it is that medicine
is meant to serve. No more in medicine than in statecraft did Franklin view
things narrowly or discuss them dogmatically. He knew too much for that, was
too widely experienced, too tolerant. This comprehension and sound sense, this
conviction that was always open to new knowledge breathe through a private
comment on mesmerism, that exceedingly popular French doctrine from which,
like electricity in its youth, all things were expected. None of the cures said to
have been effected by mesmerism, Franklin pointed out, had come under his
observation, and so he could express no opinion; but

> there being so many Disorders which cure themselves, and such a Disposition in Man-
> kind to deceive themselves and one another on these Occasions; and the living long
> having given me frequent Opportunities of seeing certain Remedies cry'd up as curing
> every thing and yet soon after totally laid aside as useless, I cannot but fear that the
> Expectation of great Advantage from this new Method of treating Diseases, will prove
> a Delusion. That Delusion may however in some cases be of use while it lasts. There
> are in every great rich City, a Number of Persons who are never in health, because
> they are fond of Medicines and always taking them, whereby they derange the natural
> Functions, and hurt their Constitutions. If these People can be persuaded to forbear their
> Drugs in Expectation of being cured by only the Physicians' Finger or an Iron Rod
> pointing at them, they may possibly find good Effects tho' they mistake the Cause.

DR. JAMES SMITH AND THE PUBLIC ENCOURAGEMENT FOR VACCINATION FOR SMALLPOX

The story of the introduction and spread of vaccination for smallpox is an interesting chapter in the history of American medicine and public health. Brought to the United States in 1800, this new defense against the disease, superseding inoculation, was spread quickly through the country from several cities and was soon practiced by numerous physicians. The medical men who did this service were for the most part undistinguished practitioners, who grasped, however, the significance of Jenner's discovery and were inspired, some of them, with a kind of zeal for it. Comprehending their task as nothing short of overcoming the popular inertia and lack of appreciation of preventive medicine and of vaccinating the entire population, a few of the more forward-looking physicians established private and semiprivate agencies to dispense vaccine and sought the encouragement of government in their labors. Such a one was Dr. James Smith, who devoted the best part of his thought and energy for more than twenty years to the cause of vaccination and who, as United States agent of vaccination, helped to spread knowledge of its usefulness through the country.

Dr. Smith was born in Elkton, Maryland, in 1771 and was educated at Dickinson College in Carlisle, Pennsylvania, from which he was graduated in 1792.[1] He then went to Philadelphia, where he probably attended medical lectures at the University of Pennsylvania and where he studied under Dr. Benjamin Rush, with whom he maintained a cordial personal and professional relation until the latter's death. Upon the completion of his formal medical studies, Smith opened an office for the practice of medicine in Baltimore. Here, as early as 1797, he began to reveal that almost overweening solicitude for the public health and its improvement which was the mainspring of his life. During the yellow fever epidemic in Baltimore in that year, Dr. Smith served as one of the two physicians assigned by the Board of Health to attend the encampment established on the outskirts of the city for the victims of the plague. Some of the facts which came within his knowledge Smith communicated privately to Dr. Rush, who gave them to the press. The Baltimore papers, jealous of the reputation of their city, denounced the facts as a libel and the Board of Health flatly denied that the fever was abroad.[2] This was Smith's first encounter with the Board. Three years later, during a recurrence of the yellow fever, Smith opened his house to sufferers and under the pseudonym of "Humanitas" addressed a series of letters to the press, arraigning the members of the Board of Health for ignorant and negligent conduct during the epidemic and proposing a reconstitution of the Board with a more vigorous personnel and more extensive powers. Warned by the Board to be cautious how he meddled in public affairs, Smith retorted with a ringing declaration that he was "determined to support the *truth*, and defend the cause of injured humanity; tho' thousands of you should rise up against it."[3] Smith's forthright attack on men and measures which he believed hurtful to the public health, his resort to the public press, and his assumption of superior knowledge and virtue were characteristic of the man and were destined to win him the hostility of the public health authorities and to alienate not a few private practitioners.

Meanwhile, in 1800, Dr. Smith was named resident physician of the Baltimore City and County Almshouse and in the following year he helped organize and became one of the attending physicians of the Baltimore General Dispensary. It was at the Almshouse on May 1, 1801, that he performed his first vaccination for smallpox.

Prior to the discovery of vaccination, protection against the almost universal and seemingly inevitable smallpox could be secured only by inoculation with virus from a mild case of the disease. This method, widely adopted in England and America in the second quarter of the eighteenth century, was rarely fatal and succeeded in reducing greatly the mortality from the smallpox. In not a few cases, however, the disease took effect severely and in none were its disfiguring effects avoided. Something of the physical ordeal of inoculation is suggested by the experience of William Pynchon, of Salem, Massachusetts, who sought protection against smallpox in 1776. In his diary he describes the doses of "powders," senna, and salts which were prescribed to aid the progress of the disease, the pains in head and limbs, the vomiting, loss of appetite, and general weakness, which succeeded the operation.[4] Furthermore, each inoculated person became for a period a source of infection from which the disease in its most virulent form might spread. This danger indeed was so great that inoculation constituted a threat to the public health less serious only than a visitation of the smallpox itself.[5]

The dangers and inconveniences of inoculation vaccination promised to avoid, and large numbers of medical men at once adopted this new means of security from smallpox. Throughout the world in the next few years, in consequence, benevolent monarchs, public-spirited physicians and philanthropists, and practitioners with an eye to profit established public and private institutions for general vaccination.[6] Laymen, accordingly, quickly learned of vaccination and the promise it held of protection from smallpox; but ignorance, prejudice, and procrastination were obstacles to an immediate general acceptance of the new method. "It has often happened to families who have been accidentally exposed to the contagion of the small pox," Dr. Smith once wrote, "that in the moment of their greatest danger they have searched in vain for a small portion of vaccine matter, to relieve them from their distressing apprehensions. Many have sent messenger after messenger to procure this remedy, and one express after another, in the greatest precipitation, and sometimes to very distant places, without being able to find it; until, at length, they have been compelled, at the risque of their lives and to the great annoyance of their neighbours to recur to the old mode of inoculating for the small pox."[7] This tendency to put off vaccination until smallpox itself appeared, this lack of appreciation of preventive medicine, was perhaps the most formidable enemy of the new method. There were others. Some doctors and many laymen clung to the old way through mental inertia. Other persons defended inoculation because it meant their livelihood: quacks in Philadelphia, it was charged in 1805, were deliberately inoculating with smallpox, under the guise of vaccinating, in order to discredit vaccination. Even religious scruples were played upon by the opponents of vaccination, who searched the Bible to prove the impiety of giving healthy men the disease of a beast.[8]

The year after Jenner announced his discovery a copy of his paper reached Dr. Benjamin Waterhouse, of Cambridge, Massachusetts. At once Waterhouse sent to England for vaccine and in July, 1800, he performed on his son the first vaccination for smallpox in America. At about the same time Dr. John Crawford, of Baltimore, received some vaccine from England, but his operations were not successful. Some months later a fresh supply of vaccine was sent to Baltimore, where it came into the hands of Dr. Smith. He, on May 1, 1801, in the Baltimore Almshouse, vaccinated a seven-year-old girl, Nancy Malcum, and during the next few weeks tried the "Cow Pox matter from England," as he wrote Rush, on several more pauper babies and children "with apparent & promising success." Although Dr. Smith performed the vaccinations in a public manner, kept records of his cases which he invited the physicians of Baltimore to examine, and offered them vaccine to use, none could be induced to vaccinate except in the Almshouse. To destroy the professional and popular suspicion of vaccination Dr. Smith published in December an unvarnished account of the summer's work. Frankly stating what he believed were the objections to the use of the cowpox, he expressed the conclusion that nevertheless vaccination for the smallpox was safer and easier than inoculation. The next year the Medical and Chirurgical Faculty of Maryland endorsed vaccination.[9]

Growing increasingly confident of the power of vaccination and realizing what it meant for the improvement of public health, Smith soon concluded that some agency should be established to preserve pure vaccine and make it more widely available. Possibly he was moved also, a young practitioner, by the desire to increase his income by becoming a vaccinator. At any rate, on March 25, 1802, with the approval of the mayor of Baltimore, the trustees of the poor of Baltimore County, and twenty-two professional colleagues, Smith opened at his home a vaccine institution, where vaccine would be preserved and distributed free of charge to such poor persons as were recommended by the subscribers to the institution. Others, of course, might be vaccinated upon payment of the usual fee. This was the first institution of its kind in the United States; but almost simultaneously other physicians in other communities, arriving at similar conclusions concerning the need of vaccination, were setting up similar institutions.[10] Tirelessly propagandizing the new discovery, vaccinating the poor and others, supplying vaccine to other physicians, Smith carried on his work with confidence and enthusiasm. His first-born son he named Edward Jenner and he vaccinated the infant when twenty-three days old. Twenty years later, his zeal in the cause of vaccination undimmed, he was to beg the mother of a girl baby whose life the 'kine pock' had saved to rename the infant Vaccina. In the next few years Smith was increasingly absorbed by the work of the vaccine institution and, as an increasing number of physicians and even some private persons applied to it for vaccine, its usefulness began to extend beyond Baltimore into the neighboring counties.

By 1809 Dr. Smith had come to the conclusion that his vaccine institution should be placed on a permanent, public, and state-wide basis. He thought it wrong, he said, that the benefit of vaccination should not be available to all without charge. Furthermore the demands of a growing family forbade him to give more attention to the work of the institution, whose increasing scope and functions had already made him relinquish some of his practice. Accordingly, in May, 1809, Dr. Smith petitioned the Maryland legislature to establish the vaccine institution as a state agency, which should preserve pure vaccine and supply it free of charge to every physician or other citizen of the state who might apply for it. For his services Smith asked $1,000 a year. The assembly, adopting instead a method which would cost the state nothing, authorized a lottery to raise not more than $30,000 "for the preservation and distribution of the vaccine matter, for the use of the citizens of this state." In return Dr. Smith was required to procure, preserve, and distribute vaccine, with directions for its use, to any citizen of the state, for a period of six years. He was thus obligated to serve as vaccine agent for the state of Maryland, with such compensation as he might be able to realize from the lottery. The managers of the vaccine agency lottery might not have done badly, however, had not the assembly at the same session authorized another more attractive lottery. Temporarily abandoned in consequence of this, Smith's lottery was finally drawn in 1812, when $12,797.20 were realized by the agency.[11]

In his effort to dispose of tickets in the lottery Dr. Smith turned to the Pennsylvania legislature. Pointing out that many persons in the western counties of that commonwealth resorted to Baltimore for vaccine, he asked permission to sell tickets in Pennsylvania, offering in return to supply the citizens of that state with pure vaccine for a period of six years. Although the lower house had less than a year before gone on record against vaccinating the poor at public expense and against prohibiting inoculation, the senate received Dr. Smith's memorial cordially. "To watch over the health and protect the lives of her citizens, appears to be most indispensably the duty of every wise government," the senate committee asserted, endorsing his plan as the most competent yet suggested to attain the grand object of security from the smallpox. Accordingly a bill was recommended to establish, for six years, two vaccine institutions, one at Philadelphia and one at Pittsburgh, under the authority and at the expense of the Commonwealth, and to name Dr. Smith an additional vaccine agent for the accommodation of those who had easier access to Baltimore. Smith traveled to Lancaster to make personal appeals to the legislators, but the bill, oddly enough, passed the house by a single vote, but was lost in the senate by two votes.[12]

Undiscouraged by the unsatisfactory nature of the law designating him vaccine agent of Maryland and by the rejection of his proposal by the Pennsylvania legislature, Dr. Smith in 1811 carried his plan to the federal Congress, offering to supply the inhabitants of the District of Columbia with vaccine. This first memorial was followed by a circular letter to the members of Congress in which Smith further offered to examine the vaccination scabs of any citizen of the United States to determine whether the operation had been successful, and to preserve vaccine for distribution to physicians and other persons throughout the United States. Although he hoped for a salary for his services, Smith expressed his willingness to undertake the office without compensation. By an act of February 27, 1813, Congress authorized the President "to appoint an agent to preserve the genuine vaccine matter, and to furnish the same to any citizen of the United States, whenever it may be applied for, through the medium of the post office," and further granted the vaccine agent the privilege of receiving and sending, postage free, letters and packages "containing vaccine matter, or relating to the subject of vaccination." There was no provision for compensation. Under the terms of this law President Madison appointed Dr. Smith United States vaccine agent.[13]

Just a year later the Virginia assembly authorized the governor of that commonwealth to contract with the national vaccine agent or any other person "to furnish the citizens of this commonwealth, applying for the same, through the medium of the post office, or in any other way, with genuine vaccine matter, and directions how to use it, free of any fee, charge, or expense whatsoever." Smith was accordingly appointed state vaccine agent for Virginia, with a compensation fixed at $600 a year.[14]

Dr. Smith was now United States vaccine agent and vaccine agent for Maryland and Virginia as well. During the thirteen years that he held one or more of these posts he occupied a unique position in American medicine and public health and had ample opportunity to render service to communities stricken or threatened by the smallpox and to inspire confidence in vaccination. The laws under which he operated required him to preserve vaccine; to Marylanders and Virginians he must distribute it free of charge, while of other citizens he might and usually did ask a fee. But Dr. Smith was at bottom a philanthropist and was never one to restrict his sense of duty to the public to the narrow terms of legislative acts. With a generous hand he supplied vaccine to the West Indies and South America as well as to all parts of the United States and often waived his fees; he sent out agents to vaccinate and propagandize in the western states and territories; and he appointed deputies throughout the land to press the cause locally. During the War of 1812 he supplied vaccine to the surgeons of the Army and the Navy. When the smallpox threatened several sections of the country in 1816, he mailed vaccine to his agents and to postmasters unsolicited, and was flattered to learn that in some cases the vaccine arrived before the disease. As national vaccine agent he employed twenty agents to travel through the country and these were estimated to have given 6750 days' service gratis and to have vaccinated upwards of 100,000 persons in the gigantic and sometimes dramatic war on the smallpox. When the Maryland act expired in 1816 and when he was removed from his national office in 1822, Dr. Smith hastened to assure the public by notices in the press that he still preserved pure vaccine as always for their protection. Whatever criticism can be made of Dr. Smith personally and even of his conduct of the vaccine agency, it can hardly be denied that he fulfilled the obligations that he undertook and that, as he himself said, he incurred "many heavy expenses, for which I never could expect to receive any pecuniary, or other reward than the satisfaction to be experienced from preventing the suffering or destruction of our fellow creatures by the smallpox."[15]

The vaccine agency, it will be seen, rested upon two principles. The first was that pure vaccine must be preserved at some known central source of supply from which it might be readily obtained whenever needed. The second principle underlying Smith's vaccine agency was that vaccination might be practiced safely by any person of average intelligence and education. To these principles Smith clung tenaciously, and upon each, as it fell out, were hung an argument and a charge that were to prove his undoing.

Individual practitioners, Dr. Smith correctly saw, could not preserve vaccine in its freshness over the long periods of time when their communities were free of smallpox; nor ought threatened areas be forced to appeal from one doctor to another until at last one was found with a supply of vaccine.[16] Other physicians, by establishing their vaccine institutions, had reached like conclusions; but Smith was the first to see that in this matter the support of government was desirable if not necessary, and his institution had been named of all others the national agency. Dr. Smith's position under the Act of 1813 was indeed vulnerable, for he was thereby designated a public agent, yet drew his income from fees charged those citizens whom it was his duty to serve. The approval of Smith's institution, which his appointment as vaccine agent implied, undoubtedly brought him more business, and the privilege of franking the letters and parcels of the institution gave him an advantage over other doctors. His rivals found it easy to charge that they were unable to secure vaccine from him, but the charge was false; and they attacked the agency as an unwarrantable monopoly, but this was at least debatable. The truth of the matter for many of them seems to be that they were irritated by his authority and jealous of his success.

But there were honester doubts of the principle of domestic vaccination, to use Professor Welch's term. Private gentlemen, Dr. Smith assured the public in 1816, might vaccinate themselves and families "with as much safety and with the same certainty of success, as if the undersigned or any other vaccinator should have performed the operation for them";[17] and to the citizens of Maryland and Virginia and of the United States generally during his service as vaccine agent, he supplied vaccine with printed directions for applying it. Legislative assemblies which approved Smith's memorials endorsed this principle: the practice of vaccination, agreed a committee of the Pennsylvania Senate, was so well understood that "intelligent persons of every profession are as adequate to it as the most learned of the [medical] faculty themselves."[18] But it was Smith's insistence that the services of a physician were not necessary in vaccination that aroused not a little of the enmity toward him displayed by professional colleagues. And it is also likely that the results of vaccinations performed by untrained persons sometimes discredited the method.

During the years that Smith was vaccine agent several local epidemics of the smallpox of varying intensity broke out. They reveal his methods. In March, 1810, informed that the disease had appeared in northern Baltimore County and that those previously vaccinated were succumbing to smallpox and were in consequence hostile to vaccination, Dr. Smith made a personal visit to the infected region and traced the trouble to his satisfaction to the use of impure vaccine. Calling a general meeting of the citizens, he stated the facts, personally vaccinated some, and left fresh vaccine with directions for its use. "The most happy results ensued from these proceedings," he wrote with pardonable pride afterwards, "the public confidence was restored in vaccination, and the small pox contagion was extirpated from among the people, affording me the satisfaction to have secured with my own hand, nearly one thousand of the citizens of Maryland and Pennsylvania from the danger to which they has been exposed." Similar methods of personal visitation, public meetings, and general vaccination were employed by Smith to avert a threatened outbreak in Calvert County, Maryland, in 1812, and to extinguish an incipient epidemic at Elk Ridge, Maryland, five years later

In Baltimore city the disease lent itself to more methodical and unremitting treatment under Smith's personal direction. A mild threat of smallpox in the city in 1810 was stamped out by Dr. Smith and a temporary vaccination society which he organized for the purpose. The next winter, however, the disease appeared again and had struck down seven persons before Smith, who had been absent from the city, could organize against it. At once sounding the alarm, he offered to examine all vaccination marks to determine their genuineness and to distribute vaccine gratis to all who might apply. For thus giving public notice of the danger which threatened the city, Dr. Smith was attacked, as his account of the yellow fever had been attacked fifteen years before, for injuring the reputation of the city and he was most viciously charged with spreading the alarm in order to make business for the vaccine institution. "The columns of our newspapers," he wrote afterwards, "soon became swelled with criticisms; and learned doctors spent their time in abusing me, instead of exercising their talents in proper efforts to extinguish the contagion which was afloat in our city." Having a start on the vaccine agent, the disease spread with uncommon speed and struck terror into the city. The Vaccine Society was reorganized with Smith as secretary, and thirty-eight physicians of the medical faculty offered to vaccinate gratuitously all who might apply. In the two years 1811 and 1812, 336 persons died of smallpox in Baltimore. When the disease broke out again in 1816 there was no delay in resorting to vaccination and only two deaths occurred.[19]

In 1816 and 1817 Dr. Smith appealed again to Congress to enact a vaccination law in the terms originally asked; that is, to have the vaccine matter supplied free of charge to every citizen of the United States who might ask for it and to compensate the agent. In his first memorial, dated January 15, 1816, Smith further asked that every vaccinating physician be required to keep records of every case, which should be forwarded to, and preserved by, the United States vaccine agent. This requirement, designed partly to protect the public from illiterate vaccinators, suggests that Smith realized—though he never publicly admitted as much—that domestic vaccination was liable to be, and had in fact been, abused by the ignorant. In his second memorial, dated December 6 of the same year, to meet constitutional objections Dr. Smith suggested that the vaccine agent be required to supply vaccine to the surgeons of the Army and the Navy. The suggestions of these memorials were incorporated into bills, which, in general, required that vaccine, with instructions for its use, be distributed gratis to the surgeons of the Army and the Navy and to all citizens of the United States, and granted the United States vaccine agent an annual compensation of $1500. In the debates the opposition argued that the proposal was an unconstitutional invasion of a field in which the states were competent to act and that it was unwise to encourage untrained persons to perform such operations. Supporters of the measure replied that the bill was within the power of Congress to enact, since it required the vaccine agent to perform certain duties for the Army and the Navy and since, further, the Constitution expressly charged Congress with responsibility to provide for the general welfare, which vaccination most certainly promoted. The first bill, however, never came to a vote; the second was defeated.[20]

In the next year, 1818, Smith sought to meet the constitutional objections to his plan and accordingly prayed that vaccine matter be supplied to the Army and the Navy, the District of Columbia, and other territories under the control of the Federal Government. Congress, although testifying their confidence in vaccination and their approbation of the manner in which Dr. Smith had conducted his office, replied that the surgeons of the Army and the Navy were competent to preserve such vaccine as they might need, without additional expense to the Government.[21]

With the Federal Government thus declining to establish the vaccine institution on any sort of national basis, with the Maryland legislature taking no action to renew Smith's commission as state vaccine agent, which had expired in 1816, and with the govenor of Virginia in 1818 appointing a citizen as vaccine agent of that commonwealth,[22] Dr. Smith knew that if the work of his vaccine institution was to be done on the scale projected, it must be with the support of private individuals. Accordingly, on February 26, 1818, he issued a public appeal for funds for a national vaccine institution to preserve pure vaccine and to supply it with directions for its use, free of charge, to all who might apply for it. By the terms set forth in the prospectus, subscribers to the institution were to receive vaccine as often as they applied for it until 1823, or, upon the final establishment of the institution, forever thereafter; as soon as funds warranted, a permanent building was to be erected in the city of Washington for the accommodation of the institution and the remainder of the funds were to be invested in government bonds; and the institution was to "be under the sole direction and control of the undersigned, during his life, should the same be convenient to him." A subsequent address to the public on the subject stated that the institution would not be permanently established until $40,000 were subscribed, that subagents would be named in every county subscribing $200 or more, and that the director of the institution was to be appointed by the President of the United States and responsible to a board of trustees, whose successors, under the terms of the bill brought in, should be appointed by the President.[23]

In less than two years $26,000 were subscribed, an organization was effected, and the managers submitted a memorial to Congress praying to be incorporated. It was "of essential importance" to the Army and the Navy, which now required vaccination, and to the citizens of the country generally, declared the memorialists, "that some central and responsible institution should be established wherein an uninterrupted supply of the genuine matter should be maintained, and from which it ought to be regularly dispensed, on the most free and liberal terms possible, to all who want it." The act of incorporation passed the House after some delay, but it died in the Senate.[24]

Although Smith was unable to secure the patronage of Congress for his National Vaccine Institution, he was still able to carry on its work. Popular confidence in vaccination and in the projected institution had not, it seems, been measurably shaken by the repeated rejection of Smith's memorials and petitions; subscriptions for the endowment of the proposed institution continued to come in, and physicians and citizens resorted to Smith for vaccine as formerly. There was every expectation that the required sum would soon be subscribed and that the National Vaccine Institution would be at last permanently though privately established. This prospect, however, was destroyed by Dr. Smith's conduct in the Baltimore smallpox epidemic of 1821-22 and by his responsibility for the tragic affair known as the Tarborough accident.

Imported from Liverpool, the smallpox quickly spread through Baltimore during the late summer of 1821 and there were several cases in the city when, late in September, Dr. Smith learned that his old enemy was abroad again. The facts of the incipient epidemic, together with a supply of vaccine, Dr. Smith on September 30 sent the physicians of the city. But the most astounding and distressing fact about the new outbreak was that one of the victims was a girl whom Smith himself had vaccinated as an infant some years before. The conclusion seemed inescapable: vaccination was no sure preventive of smallpox. To the press the next day Smith communicated this startling reversal of opinion concerning vaccination.[25] No matter how carefully he might word his statement, the damage was done. The public knew only that smallpox was abroad and that vaccination was no sure defense against it.

The death toll from the disease mounted steadily during the next two months, until finally in December the Medical and Chirurgical Faculty, at Smith's suggestion, in a statement expressing Smith's new view of the limitations of vaccination, called for action. Accordingly, by public ordinance physicians were appointed to vaccinate the poor of the city and to induce all others to submit to the operation. Private activity supplemented the public efforts. In January the Vaccine Society was reorganized with Dr. Smith, who was now, it seems, returning to his former confidence in vaccination, as secretary; and, adopting the methods which proved so successful in the epidemic of 1812, its agents performed nearly 1000 vaccinations, 700 of them gratuitously. These efforts prevailed and the epidemic was suppressed, but not until more than 200 persons had died.[26]

During the epidemic Dr. Smith had endeavored to restore a measure of public confidence in vaccination by republishing an account of the exposure of his five children, all vaccinated in infancy, to a virulent case of smallpox;[27] but Smith's public letter of October 1 had had too complete an effect. What shreds of confidence may have survived were destroyed in the course of his dispute with Dr. Nathaniel Potter, of the University of Maryland medical faculty. Denying Dr. Potter's contention that only by repeated vaccination could permanent immunity be secured, Smith wrote, "I do not know who would not rather have the inoculated smallpox at once—than suffer such everlasting and uncertain repetitions of vaccination as you propose."[28] It was a strange spectacle indeed to see Dr. James Smith, after twenty years' devotion to vaccination, not only doubting the efficacy of the cow pox, but even seeming to condone inoculation. The medical profession did not remain silent, but none could have taken the same satisfaction from Smith's plight which his Baltimore rivals and the Baltimore Board of Health so evidently enjoyed.[29]

While the smallpox and the paper war over it were continuing in Baltimore, Smith was confronted by another event which further shook his and the public's confidence in vaccination and was the immediate occasion of Smith's removal from the office of United States vaccine agent and the final destruction of the office itself. The details of the Tarborough affair are not clear but the facts can be stated broadly.[30] About November 1, 1821, Dr. Smith prepared an envelope for Dr. John F. Ward, recently appointed a deputy agent of the National Vaccine Institution in Tarborough, N. C., containing, as Smith believed, a personal letter and some vaccine put up between glass. Late in December Ward wrote Dr. Smith explaining that the vaccine had produced a reaction not unlike smallpox itself. Two weeks later Smith learned definitely that the persons whom Ward had vaccinated had indeed been infected with the smallpox and that several deaths had resulted. Smith was having trouble enough. Vaccination, the Baltimore epidemic seemed to show, was not infallible protection against the disease; now the North Carolina experience appeared to suggest that vaccine might produce smallpox itself. Some physicians began to resort to inoculation. That at least was certain.

Thoroughly alarmed, without waiting to learn all the facts, Smith published a letter in which he set forth what he knew and attempted to explain what had happened. Perhaps, he suggested, smallpox contagion had clung to his person as he prepared the vaccine; or, he thought, the genuine cow pox was so nearly like smallpox that when the disease becomes epidemic "it intermixes with the vaccine matter by a natural process"; perhaps the same person may be a carrier of both smallpox and cow pox; finally he expressed his conjecture that cow pox, which furnished vaccine one day, may undergo such changes as in a few days to furnish matter capable of producing smallpox. These speculations, however, were quickly denounced by physicians and public health authorities as issued "for the inexcusable purpose of justifying an unfortunate mistake."[31]

Hardly had this ill-considered letter appeared when the facts came from North Carolina. The vaccine was not vaccine crusts at all, but smallpox scabs. Wrapped in a piece of paper marked "Variol," they had been sent by some chance to Ward and he had ignorantly used them in vaccinating the community. This new development Smith communicated at once to the Speaker of the House of Representatives, where the matter was now under discussion. Nothing was wrong with the vaccine, Smith explained; a mistake had happened this once but "there is no danger that the like will ever occur again."[32] Smith's enemies, however, preferred to believe that his first explanation had been made to avoid the responsibility for his conduct; that his second was written only because the first was unacceptable.

In Congress Hutchins G. Burton, representative from North Carolina, demanded the repeal of the law under which Smith had been appointed vaccine agent. A committee friendly to Smith reported its entire confidence in vaccination as a preventive of smallpox, expressed itself as "decidedly of opinion" that vaccination should be performed only by trained physicians, and concluded by those charged with the execution of the act, that is, by removal from office, no change in the law should be made. But Mr. Burton was not to be thus easily dissuaded from his purpose. Ten men, he declaimed, had lost their lives by the act of a man who styled himself an agent of the United States and a law of the United States had put it in his power to do this irreparable injury. Burton was named chairman of a select committee to consider the act. On April 13 the committee presented its report recommending repeal. The regulation of the public health, the committee asserted in the first place, is a police question which appertains peculiarly "to the municipal authorities in the several states, and which must, of necessity, be finally committed to the management and discretion of professional men possessing the confidence of the community." The privilege of franking letters, the committee went on, and of acquiring wealth by levying a fee for the vaccine, "affords an instance of monopoly as repugnant to the spirit of our political institutions as it is to the character of the medical profession, which, for public spirited and active benevolence, is too well established to require auxiliaries of this description in the performance of its duties." Finally, the committee thought, a single agent was not sufficient to meet the demands for vaccine from all sections of the country. Around these ideas and the specific instance of Smith's conduct in the Tarborough affair the debate revolved. Inasmuch as Smith had been removed from his office by the President on April 10, the question was one of policy alone. Nonetheless, Burton attacked Smith's good faith, while Mr. Wright came to the agency's defense, asking whether the smallpox was not "more likely to have been introduced by the North Carolina doctors, whose interest it was to have the people as sick as they could be." Despite the strong defense of Lewis Condict, of New Jersey, and John Floyd, of Virginia, both professional medical men, the act of repeal became a law on May 4.[33] In Baltimore *Niles' Weekly Register* rejoiced in the destruction of the agency: vaccination "would have succeeded far better, if less reliance had been placed on the agent and more on those whose business it is to attend to and mark the progress of that remedy."[34]

The Congressional action, which seemed to imply acceptance of Burton's charges against him and a denial of value to the agency left Smith resentful. It is to this period and possibly to this spirit that Smith's patenting of his method of sending vaccine through the mails belongs.[35] Still, he continued his work as formerly, immediately announcing in the press that he continued to preserve the vaccine matter as before and that his efforts were unabated to establish the National Vaccine Institution as originally proposed. "I can assure the public," he declared in a public notice—for he had returned to his original view of the permanent efficacy of vaccination—"that when perfect kine pock matter is used, and the vaccine process is suffered to terminate without interruption, vaccination is a sure preventive of the small pox."[36] Private subscriptions enabled the work of the National Vaccine Institution to continue for a time, but by the end of 1823 the funds were exhausted and Smith was, he confessed, "in consequence obliged to retire in some measure, from the contest in which he had been so long and so successfully engaged in opposing the progress of the small pox." Meanwhile, of course, vaccine institutions were being established in other parts of the country, so that there was increasingly less need to resort to Baltimore. It was doubtless so that he might carry on that in this year Dr. Smith again prayed the aid of Congress for the National Vaccine Institution, but without success. In 1824 and again in 1825, pointing to the alarming increase of smallpox in the country, he presented memorials praying in the first for the reappointment of a central vaccine agent, with deputies in each congressional district and with a fixed compensation, and in the second for a renewal of the franking privilege for his institution. Friendly committees approved in both instances, but the bills they presented never came to a vote.[37]

Coupled with Smith's continued exertions on behalf of vaccination was his desire to clear himself of the charge of negligence in the Tarborough accident. In March, 1822, while the matter was still under Congressional investigation, he began to publish *The Vaccine Inquirer*, which reprinted his various public letters and notices on vaccination and contained especially the documents relating to the Tarborough case. In his memorials to Congress in 1824 and 1825 Dr. Smith reviewed his part in the affair and offered a new reconstruction of the unhappy events. A reconsideration of all the facts led Dr. Smith to conclude that his letter to Dr. Ward had been deliberately tampered with by someone intent on destroying him. Smith had always charged that a considerable body of the medical profession was hostile to him and his institution and that they had employed the Tarborough incident as a means to destroy him; but whether this new and almost incredible charge was true it is impossible now to say. The Congressional committees wisely refrained from endorsing Smith's view of the matter. One, however, gave its thought that there was more reason to impute the accident to "some secret hand not responsible" than to Smith; while a second expressed what must probably be the last word on the subject: "The Committee see no ground to impute to Doctor Smith any want of skill, or of care and attention, in conducting the vaccine agency, and much less of any evil design to propagate the pestilence, as has been charged upon him. There yet remains some obscurity as to the facts of the case."[38]

Hardly had he secured this vindication than Smith was engaged in a bitter quarrel with the Baltimore Board of Health over the relative value of vaccination and quarantine as defenses against smallpox. With all his former energy he insisted that vaccination was the only sure preventive and protection; quarantine laws "are good for very little, and of no use, as a means of preventing the introduction of the small-pox"; and further, he added, passing over to personalities, the officers of the Board of Health were neither faithful nor competent to their duty. The Board had a defense equal to the attack. "What motives," one of its members wished to know, "can prompt Dr. Smith to hang about small pox patients, like a preying vulture? We know of no more ready way of spreading the disease, than by the unnecessary and presumptuous interference of Dr. Smith, with what does not concern him. As it is his interest, may it not be his intention, in keeping up this intercourse with the sick, to spread the disease?"[39] In this blast and counter-blast Dr. Smith, his best work for vaccination done, it seems, passed out of the history of medicine and public health in Baltimore.

Dr. Smith died at Pikesville, Maryland, on June 12, 1841, but his death was unnoticed by the medical journals or by the press of the city in whose welfare, as he had written Dr. Rush more than forty years before, he felt himself closely interested and whose health and prosperity he ever viewed with pleasure. Certainly he deserved little extended notice as a scientist, for, although he apparently kept his records carefully, he cannot be said to have learned all they had to teach him of vaccination.[40] An an experimentalist, for example, might have profited much by the discovery that a person once vaccinated may subsequently be liable to smallpox, but Smith allowed himself to be frightened from determining the meaning of this fact by the fury of his enemies and the testimonies of his friends.

Moreover Dr. Smith had serious limitations as a public health officer. Though the head of a vaccine institution for twenty years, with an uncharted field to develop, with the approval of two states and the federal government, with the beginnings of a national reputation and the likelihood of national support, Smith built nothing that survived him. Essentially a moralist, to him laws and regulations meant little, character everything. His proposals for revamping the Baltimore Board of Health, for example, and for his own National Vaccine Institution were all of them loosely drawn and rested in the end for their effective execution on the personality of the appointees, of the appointee, rather. For Smith was the Vaccine Institution, a kind of self-appointed physician-at-large to the nation; and when he retired there was no successor. If Dr. Smith organized nothing, this was doubtless because he was unable or unwilling to share responsibility for the Institution, unwilling to share credit for its work. Of his own character, honest, tireless, humane, Smith had no doubt and, expecting others to be not otherwise, he was often impatient with them and uncooperative. He never made the slightest effort, for example, to cooperate with the Baltimore health authorities. Such a spirit in him grew and as a result, as well as under the lash of his enemies, he came finally, it seems, to believe himself wiser and more unselfish than others; he came to resent criticism; and he lost opportunities to profit from the experience of others. He might profitably have considered, for example, Dr. Potter's suggestion that only by repeated vaccination can permanent immunity be obtained, and he was only stubborn when he ascribed the misfortunes of vaccination in part to ignorant and unskilful vaccinators and as often insisted that any man is competent to vaccinate any other.

Even Dr. Smith's honesty and directness lay near the bottom of the destruction of his career. Seemingly incapable of verifying his ideas by testing them, he printed hypotheses as conclusions, doing harm as well as good. It was an honest way, to keep the public acquainted with the progress of his thought, and it inspired the confidence which allowed him in the early days of his work to vaccinate whole communities; but in 1821 it spread, albeit unwittingly, distrust and as much alarm and confusion as the smallpox itself. Dr. Smith might have been cautious, yet have concealed nothing, and caution might have spared vaccination some of its discredit and Smith the destruction of his reputation.

When all this is said, however, it still remains to say that in the history of vaccination in America, in the larger history of preventive medicine and the public health, and in the history of humanitarian service, Dr. James Smith occupies a merited place. At very least, he and his appointed agents, to say nothing of all others who obtained vaccine from him, gave tens of thousands of Americans protection from smallpox. But more than this, he saw clearly that vaccine must be preserved in some central and known place from which it might be distributed as needed; and, though, with his age, he would never have dreamed of making vaccination compulsory, he realized that government must have some responsibility for this public health measure. Despite prejudice and constitutional objections, his contemporaries and successors came to accept this view of the matter.[41] For his theory of domestic vaccination, on the other hand, whatever the theoretical merits of the case, he failed to win approval; but this was probably no great loss.

REFERENCES

1. Biographical data may be found easily in: HOWARD A. KELLY, ed., A Cyclopaedia of American Medical Biography, comprising the lives of eminent deceased physicians and surgeons from 1610 to 1910, Philadelphia and London, 1912, 2:385. EUGENE F. CORDELL, The Medical Annals of Maryland, 1799-1899, Baltimore, 1903, pp. 669, 672-74, et passim. JOHN R. QUINAN, The introduction of inoculation and vaccination into Maryland, historically considered, Maryland Medical Journal, 10:113-19, 129-33 (June 23, 30) 1883; QUINAN, Medical Annals of Baltimore from 1608 to 1880, Including Events, Men and Literature, Baltimore, 1884, pp. 22-31, 155-56. WILLIAM H. WELCH, "Vaccination," typescript address before the Baltimore City Medical Society, Nov. 4, 1932, in Medical and Chirurgical Faculty of Maryland, Library. These accounts are based largely on Smith's memorials and letters which were reprinted in A Society of Physicians, The Vaccine Inquirer: or, Miscellaneous Collections Relative to Vaccination, Baltimore, 1822-24. Smith is not listed in the Catalogue of the Medical Graduates of the University of Pennsylvania, Philadelphia, 1836.
2. Smith to Rush, Baltimore, Aug. 31, 1797. Rush MSS., Correspondence, XXIII, 116. Library Company of Philadelphia, Ridgway Branch.
3. Federal Gazette and Baltimore Daily Advertiser, Nov. 12, 13, 18, 22, Dec. 5, 12, 1800. The controversy was continued by Smith in The Additional Number to the Letters of Humanitas, together with John Hillen's William Jenkins's & Doctor M'Kenzie's letters—and other docu-

ments, relative to Polly Elliott's case: to which are added, Mr. Jesse Hollingsworth's letter—
and a reply to the same, Baltimore, Feb. 9, 1801. A copy of this rare pamphlet is in the William
H. Welch Medical Library, Baltimore.

4. FITCH EDWARD OLIVER, ed., The Diary of William Pynchon of Salem, Boston and New
York, 1890, pp. 10-18.

5. See, for example, the Virginia Act of Assembly of Dec. 21, 1792, printed in facsimile in *Annals
of Medical History*, 7:192-197, 1925. A Society for Inoculating the Poor Gratis was instituted
at Philadelphia in February, 1774, but in September the physicians of the city "agreed to inoculate no patients for the small pox during the sitting of Congress, as several of the Northern
and Southern delegates have not had that disorder." J. THOMAS SCHARF and THOMPSON
WESTCOTT, History of Philadelphia, 1609-1884, Philadelphia, 1884, 2:1476.

6. *Philadelphia Medical Museum*, 1:215, 224-25, 353-54, 401-06, 453-57, 1805. JOHN REDMAN
COXE, Practical Observations on Vaccination: or Inoculation for the Cow-Pock,
Philadelphia, 1802. This work Dr. Coxe dedicated to Jenner, and he named his son Edward
Jenner. On January 15, 1802, Dr. John Archer, Jr., wrote Dr. Coxe from Harford County,
Md., asking for some vaccine and instructions for its use (Gilbert Collection of Manuscript
Letters, 1:23. College of Physicians of Philadelphia, Library); and in the same year Dr.
Samuel Brown introduced vaccination into Louisville, Ky. (Dictionary of American Bio-
graphy, 3:152-53).

7. Memorial to the Pennsylvania Legislature, Jan. 15, 1810. *Senate Journal*, 1809-10, 201.

8. *Philadelphia Medical Museum*, 1:71, 434-40, 1805.

9. Smith to Rush, Baltimore, May 20, 1801. Rush MSS., Corres., XXII, 27; Vaccine Inquirer, pp.
16-37; Cordell, *op. cit.*, p. 46.

10. Vaccine Inquirer, pp. 16-20. This proposal is reprinted, with some biographical material, in
HELEN C. BROOKE, A proposal for a free vaccine clinic in Baltimore in 1802, Johns
Hopkins University Institute of the History of Medicine, *Bulletin*, 3:83-91, 1935.

11. SMITH, Two letters relative to the Vaccine Institution, addressed to the members of the Hon.
the General Assembly of Maryland, Baltimore, 1818, pp. 2-12; Prospectus of a permanent national vaccine institution, to be established in the city of Washington, District of Columbia,
Baltimore, 1818, pp. 11-13, 17. KILTY, HARRIS and WATKINS, comps., The Laws of
Maryland, from . . . 1799 . . . 1809, vol. 4, ch. 123.

12. *Senate Journal*, 1809-10, 199-203, 314-20; *ibid.*, 1810-11, 288; *House Journal*, 1808-1809, 815-18;
Ibid., 1810-11, 452-54, 462. Smith to Rush, Baltimore, Oct. 31, 1810. Rush MSS., Corres.,
XXIII, 119. The Pennsylvania legislature in the next year also rejected the petitions of Dr.
Samuel Agnew for aid in establishing a vaccine agency at Harrisburg. *House Journal*,
1811-12, 210-11; *ibid.*, 1812-13, 67-69, 171-72, 319-20.

13. Vaccine Inquirer, pp. 41-45. To the Honble. the Senate and House of Representatives of the
United States, the memorial of James Smith, agent of vaccination, Georgetown, 1816, pp.
14-15. Annals of Congress, 11 Cong. 3 sess., 839; United States Statutes at Large, 2:806-07.

14. Act of Feb. 4, 1814. Acts of Virginia, 1813-14, ch. xiv, pp. 43-44. Calendar of Virginia State
Papers and Other Manuscripts, 10:400, 410-11, 464. This law was repealed on March 6, 1821,
but re-enacted on Feb. 11, 1832. Acts of Virginia, 1820-21, ch. viii, p. 11; *ibid.*, 1831-32, ch. xxv,
pp. 25-26.

15. SMITH, Prospectus, pp. 21-29; Two letters, p. 2. American State Papers, Miscellaneous,
2:919-21. DR. ROBERT GOLDSBOROUGH, Report, Nov., 1816, MS. in Medical and Chirurgical
Faculty of Maryland, Library; notices in *Federal Gazette*, July 16, 1816, June 6, 1822;
American Volunteer, Carlisle, Pa., March 20, 1817.

16. What fearful delays this might result in is suggested by the case of Cincinnati, O. When
smallpox broke out there in 1804, "the alarmed inhabitants" appealed to Senator Smith in
Washington for vaccine; he sought it of the doctors in the capital. Unable to secure any there,
he wrote Dr. Stoughton in Burlington, N. J., but there was no vaccine in Burlington.
Stoughton wrote Dr. Rush in Philadelphia, begging him to get some if he could. W.
Stoughton to Rush, Burlington, Jan. 24, 1805. Rush MSS., Corres., XXII, 25.

17. *Federal Gazette*, July 16, 1816.

18. *Senate Journal*, 1809-10, 318.

19. SMITH, Two Letters, pp. 18-22, 29-30. (Baltimore) *American and Commercial Daily Advertiser*,

Sept. 3, 1810. QUINAN, Medical Annals, pp. 25-27. WILLIAM T. HOWARD, JR., Public Health Administration and the Natural History of Disease in Baltimore, Maryland, 1797-1920, Washington, 1924, p. 277.

20. Annals of Congress, 14 Cong. 1 sess., 719, 1408, 1455-56, 1457; ibid., 14 Cong. 2 sess., 254, 266, 361-62, 364, 468-70. SMITH, [Memorial] To the Honble, the Senate and House of Representatives. In 1818 the House passed, but the Senate rejected, a bill to extend the franking privilege to such state and territorial agents of vaccination as might be appointed. Annals of Congress, 15 Cong., 1 sess., 299, 499-500, 542, 1452.

21. SMITH, Prospectus, pp. 21-31. Annals of Congress, 15 Cong., 1 sess., 710, 846.

22. Calendar of Virginia State Papers, 10: 474, 475.

23. SMITH, Prospectus; SMITH, The National Vaccine Institution, Baltimore, July 5, 1819.

24. Am. State Papers, Misc., 2:565-67. Annals of Congress, 16 Cong., 1 sess., 858; 2 sess., 152, 242-43, 462, 471-73.

25. Federal Gazette, Oct. 2, 1821.

26. The Constitution of the Baltimore Vaccine Society, for Exterminating the Small Pox, Baltimore, 1822. HOWARD, op. cit., 55, 277. Federal Gazette, Dec. 17, 19, 1821. Report of the Health Committee, and Accompanying Documents of the Board of Physicians Appointed to Direct the Vaccination of the City, Baltimore, 1822. SMITH, Appeal to the Citizens of Baltimore in His Own Vindication, Baltimore, 1828, pp. 85-91. The title page of this last pamphlet was missing from the copy consulted in the Maryland Historical Society.

27. Niles' Weekly Register, 21:300-01 (Jan. 5) 1822. Federal Gazette, Dec. 18, 1821.

28. SMITH to Potter, Feb. 11, 1822, (Baltimore) American, Feb. 13, 1822.

29. HORATIO G. JAMESON, Some account of the small-pox which prevailed at Baltimore during the winter of 1821-22, American Medical Recorder, 5:224-56, 1822. THOMAS D. MITCHELL, A candid inquiry into the present state of vaccination, ibid., 257-68, 1822, HENRY W. DUCACHET, Strictures on the late circular addressed to the citizens of the United States by James Smith, M.D., agent of the Vaccine Institution, at Baltimore, New York Medical and Physical Journal, 1:42-53 (Jan.-March), 1822. Report of the Health Committee. DR. PATRICK MACAULAY to the editor of the National Intelligencer, Baltimore, Feb. 2, 1822, reprinted in (Baltimore) American, Feb. 15, 1822.

30. Letters and documents are reprinted in the Vaccine Inquirer, pp. 45-48, 109-44, 151-93, and in the Congressional reports cited below.

31. Report of the Health Committee.

32. Am. State Papers, Misc., 2:919.

33. Annals of Congress, 17 Cong., 1 sess., 434, 440, 351-54, 921, 1130-31, 1382, 1634-40. Am. State Papers, Misc., 2:919-21, 933-34. United States Statutes at Large, 3:677.

34. Niles' Weekly Register, 22:129 (April 27) 1822.

35. Dr. Smith's improvement consisted of moistening a fresh vaccine crust and rubbing it with a piece of glass or ivory, to which it adhered when dry, thus permitting it to "be transmitted by letter conveniently to the most distant places." The original patent, dated July 10, 1822 is in Medical and Chirurgical Faculty of Maryland Museum.

36. Federal Gazette, June 6, 1822.

37. Annals of Congress, 17 Cong., 2 sess., 577, 643; ibid., 18 Cong., 1 sess., 1428, 1739-40. House Reports, 19 Cong., 2 sess., No. 95, 3-4; Vaccine Inquirer, pp. 205-14.

38. Annals of Congress, 18 Cong., 1 sess., 1740. House Report, 19 Cong., 2 sess., No. 95.

39. SMITH, Appeal, pp. 13, 19-20, et passim.

40. For a different view of Smith as a scientist, see Brooke, loc. cit.

41. In 1827 Dr. Joseph G. Nancrede, public vaccine physician of Philadelphia, memorialized Congress to take some action to diffuse "the blessings of vaccination to the people of the United States, and, more especially, to secure its advantages to those citizens who inhabit our remote and newly settled frontiers." House Executive Documents. 20 Cong., 1 sess., No. 66. Ten years later Dr. Sylvanus Fansher, who had been associated with Waterhouse, prayed Congress to establish a permanent vaccine institution for the benefit of the army, navy, and Indian department. Senate Documents, 25, Cong., 2 sess., No. 385. In 1839 the American Journal of the Medical Sciences (24:528) endorsed a memorial of some Mercer County, Pa., physicians that vaccine be permitted to be sent through the mails postage free.

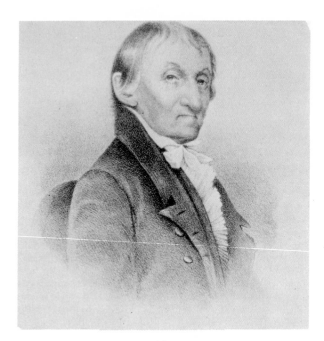

James Thacher

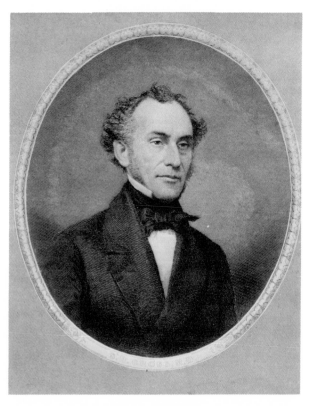

Samuel D. Gross

LIVES IN MEDICINE:
THE BIOGRAPHICAL DICTIONARIES OF THACHER, WILLIAMS, AND GROSS *

Biography has long been one of the most popular approaches to medical history. Lives have a dramatic appeal to readers which impersonal histories often lack, while non-professional historians, who have written so much medical history, are likely to view their field in terms of famous men and dramatic events and discoveries. Cushing's *Life of Sir William Osler* and Shryock's *Development of Modern Medicine* are both great books, but the former is the more representative of the bulk of medical historiography. The point is underlined by the fact that one third of all the books and articles on American medical history published between 1939 and 1960 were biographical; they exceeded the total number of those on the history of diseases, hospitals, medical education, medical sciences and specialties, public health, and the medical profession.[1]

The usefulness of biographies of course should not be decried. Until persons and events are properly identified, the course of history cannot be adequately charted. The achievements of eminent physicians and surgeons are, in fact, often landmarks in medical history; and a carefully written biography, even of a man of second rank, illustrates the principal movements in history and may in fact sometimes require the historian to modify or even abandon an accepted generalization. A picture of early American medical thought and practice based on the work and writings of Rush, Bard, Warren, and Waterhouse will be very different—and far less complete and typical—from the picture that would emerge from a study of the far greater number of undistinguished practitioners, some of

---

* Read at the Annual Dinner of the 40th annual meeting of the American Association for the History of Medicine, New Haven, Conn., April 28, 1967.

The authors and their books are: James Thacher, *American Medical Biography: or Memoirs of Eminent Physicians Who Have Flourished in America* (Boston, 1828); Stephen W. Williams, *American Medical Biography: or, Memoirs of Eminent Physicians . . . Who Have Died since the Publication of Dr. Thacher's Work on the Same Subject* (Greenfield, 1845); and Samuel D. Gross, *Lives of Eminent American Physicians and Surgeons of the Nineteenth Century* (Philadelphia, 1861).

[1] Genevieve Miller, ed., *Bibliography of the History of Medicine of the United States and Canada, 1939-1960* (Baltimore: Johns Hopkins Press, 1964).

whom were also farmers or country clergymen. These and other values appear in some of the biographical dictionaries published in the United States in the first part of the nineteenth century. For the medical historian the most important are *American Medical Biography,* 1828, by Dr. James Thacher of Plymouth, Mass.; a book of the same title, 1845, by Dr. Stephen W. Williams of Deerfield, Mass.; and *Lives of Eminent American Physicians and Surgeons of the Nineteenth Century,* 1861, by Dr. Samuel D. Gross of Philadelphia.

As their titles suggest, the two earliest books are similar in content and treatment; indeed Williams regarded his as a continuation of Thacher's. Thacher's *American Medical Biography* contained sketches of 168 physicians who had lived between the time of the first settlements and 1828, the date of its publication; and Williams' volume presented 110 biographies, principally of men who had died since the completion of Thacher's work. Gross, on the other hand, singled out a limited number —only 32—of leaders of the profession who had been in active practice during the first sixty years of the nineteenth century. While some of Thacher's and Williams' sketches were hardly more than a paragraph, Gross gave each of his subjects a full, in some cases an exhaustive, treatment. Many of Thacher's biographies and most of Williams' were more or less revisions or condensations of memorial notices or obituaries first printed in medical journals; but Gross, contemptuous in his forthright Pennsylvania-German way of glowing eulogies which, he said, concealed their subjects under flowers of rhetoric, secured original essays from authors competent to estimate the significance of their subject's achievement.

All three biographers had a common motive—to rescue from oblivion the stories of the lives of their predecessors. In doing this, they would record the history of the medical profession in America, for they believed that biography is, as Williams quoted someone as saying, the " very heart of history." They intended to serve more than piety and history, however. Sensible that the American public in the second third of the century did not esteem doctors highly, the biographers aimed to present the profession in a good light. " Physicians are called to move in a humbler sphere than clergymen, lawyers, and statesmen," Williams conceded in his preface. " Hence they are much less noticed by the great body of the people than these more prominent actors on the theatre of life. But we deny that they are less learned, useful, and good." [2] Gross put it more simply: the aim of his *Lives,* he wrote, was " to popularize

---

[2] Williams, *American Medical Biography,* pp. xiii-xiv.

the profession, and to place its services and claims more conspicuously than has yet been done, before the American people." [3] One consequence of this special motive was that both Williams and Gross gave a good many paragraphs and even pages to accounts of their subjects' final illnesses and last declarations of Christian belief. Such accounts gratified contemporary readers generally and demonstrated to a suspicious public that physicians were not an irreligious lot, as was so often charged.

Americans of the early nineteenth century seem to have been especially interested in national biography. They needed to identify the heroes of the new republic. Thus as early as 1794 the Rev. Jeremy Belknap began his *American Biography,* which was a history of America related in the lives of outstanding figures from Madoc and Columbus on. John Sanderson's *Lives of the Signers of the Declaration of Independence,* begun in 1820 on the eve of the semi-centennial of American independence, and J. T. Headley's *Washington and his Generals,* published in 1847, were other examples of this biographical approach to history. More thoughtful chroniclers appreciated the need and opportunity to record and celebrate the contributions made by many lesser persons to the establishment of the nation. William Allen prepared an excellent scholarly biographical dictionary in 1809, and Benjamin F. French published another in 1825. Meanwhile biographies limited to sections of the nation appeared. John Eliot in 1809 and Samuel L. Knapp in 1821 published volumes of biographies of New England worthies; and William L. Wirt made plans to compile a collection of lives of eminent Virginians. Thacher's *American Medical Biography* was only another example of this historico-biographical movement. What was unusual about it was that it was limited to a single profession.[4]

James Thacher (1754-1844)

James Thacher was born in 1754, the son of " a respectable farmer " of Barnstaple on Cape Cod in Massachusetts. At the age of 16 he was

---

[3] Gross, *Lives,* p. ix. Dr. John Bell of Philadelphia, who contributed a biography to Gross' work, held similar views. He rebuked his colleagues for not studying their own history enough—" the great deeds, the true heroism of our professional ancestors . . . ought to form an integral part of the history of mankind, and find their place in the brightest passages of the history of every civilized people "—and called on them to recall the memory of great doctors, partly to " impress our fellow-men, in all the walks of life, with our true position and aims." *Medical Heroism: Address before the Philadelphia County Medical Society, Delivered February 24, 1859* (Philadelphia, 1859), p. 14.

[4] Though there was no American precedent for a medical biography, Thacher might point to at least one English work—Benjamin Hutchinson's *Biographica Medica* (2 vols., London, 1799).

apprenticed to a local physician, the eccentric and unsociable Abner Hersey. His term expiring just as war broke out at Lexington and Concord in 1775, young Thacher secured appointment as a surgeon's mate in the provincial military hospital at Cambridge. He served at Ticonderoga and Albany, was surgeon to a Virginia regiment (whose officers' habits he thought " almost approached dissipation "), and ended the war at Yorktown, where he witnessed Cornwallis' surrender.[5]

The war over, Thacher settled at Plymouth, Massachusetts, where, thanks to his army experience, he soon acquired a good practice and won reputation as a skilful surgeon. He continued in active practice until he was in his 70's. To practice Thacher soon added writing—the *American New Dispensatory* in 1810, *Observations on Hydrophobia* in 1812, the *American Modern Practice* in 1817. This last contained some pages of general American medical history.

He had long been interested in history and had written several short pieces for the Massachusetts Historical Society and the American Academy of Arts and Sciences. In 1821 he commenced to write an account of his experiences in the Revolutionary War, using his journal as the basis for a narrative which was greatly extended by materials gleaned from other books and from the recollections of other veterans. The *Military Journal,* published in 1823, met with immediate success; a second edition was called for at once; and in the 20 years after Thacher's death, nine more editions were published. It remains one of the principal documentary sources for the history of the war.

Encouraged by the success of the *Military Journal,* Thacher next undertook the *American Medical Biography.* A " circular " was distributed to postmasters and others, announcing the book and soliciting assistance in collecting data on doctors, particularly " their ancestry, dates of birth and death, with the place or places of education and sphere of action; a particular detail of character or prominent traits of character, with appropriate memorials and anecdotes; to which should be added a proper notice of all publications of which they have been the authors." [6] Thacher drew on his personal knowledge of Massachusetts physicians and

[5] Williams included a biographical sketch of Thacher in his *American Medical Biography*, pp. 565-580. See also Henry R. Viets, "James Thacher and his influence on American medicine," *Virginia M. Monthly,* 1949, *8*: 384-399, and Viets' sketch in *Dictionary of American Biography*. A fuller account of Thacher, with citations of manuscript and other sources, introduces a facsimile edition of Thacher's book, published by Da Capo Press, New York, 1967.

[6] " Circular. American Medical Biography." A copy, with a note by Thacher to Isaac Goodwin, postmaster of Sterling, Mass., Jan. 25, 1826, is in Francis A. Countway Library of Medicine, Harvard Medical School.

PROPOSALS

FOR PUBLISHING THE

AMERICAN MEDICAL BIOGRAPHY,

OR

MEMOIRS OF EMINENT PHYSICIANS

WHO HAVE FLOURISHED IN AMERICA.

TO WHICH IS PREFIXED,

A SUCCINCT HISTORY OF MEDICAL SCIENCE

IN THE UNITED STATES,

FROM THE FIRST SETTLEMENT OF THE COUNTRY.

BY JAMES THACHER, M.D. M.M.S. A.A.S.

Author of the American New Dispensatory, Modern Practice of Physic, &c. &c.

It is a grateful undertaking to rescue from oblivion and transmit to posterity, the names and characters of those who have finished their career on the theatre of life and are worthy of perpetual remembrance. It was the opinion of Dr. Johnson that " no species of writing is more worthy of cultivation than biography, which, from its diversity, is capable of diffusing useful instruction in a pleasing manner to people of every condition." Perhaps no profession is more rich in this department of literature than the medical, and in none can it be applied with deeper interest or greater utility. Memoirs in detail, of those who have excelled in their professional course, not only excite a laudable emulation in the young, but furnish the aged with the consoling reflection that their own merit may not be forgotten, and that their fame will live when they are at rest. The work now to be presented to the public, will exhibit the lives of nearly two hundred physicians, forming a group of as meritorious medical characters as ever adorned any country. It will not be calculated exclusively for medical men, but will interest the attention of all classes of readers.

CONDITIONS.

1. The work will be comprised in one volume octavo, of about 600 pages, and will be printed on good paper, and well executed.
2. It will be embellished with eight or ten portraitures of eminent physicians.
3. The price to subscribers will be $ 3,50 in boards, with canvass backs.
4. Those who become accountable for six copies, will be entitled to a seventh gratis.
5. The names of the subscribers will be printed at the end of the volume, and they are requested to add their title and address for that purpose.
6. It will be put to press as soon as a sufficient number of subscribers are obtained.

☞ It is requested that subscription papers may be returned to Messrs. RICHARDSON & LORD or COTTONS & BARNARD, Boston, by the first of September next.

June 1, 1827.

Fig. 1. Thacher's " Proposals." Courtesy of the Boston Medical Library in the Francis A. Countway Library of Medicine

asked Dr. David Hosack and Dr. John W. Francis of New York, Dr. James Mease of Philadelphia, Dr. George C. Shattuck of Boston, and others for memoirs of their friends. The result was a compilation in two volumes of 168 sketches, ranging from a few lines for John Clark (d. 1676) of Rhode Island, to more than 40 pages for Samuel Bard and Benjamin Rush. The sketches were prefaced by a history of medicine and a summary of medical education in the United States which was nearly 100 pages long.

Thacher wrote to many people to get the materials for his book, and he edited them with critical judgment. The sketch of Zabdiel Boylston illustrates his carefulness. The Boylston family believed that their ancestor had been the first in London to inoculate against smallpox, and that he had there inoculated members of the royal family. These statements, a compound of truth, misapprehension, and error, were communicated to Thacher in a sketch furnished by the venerable Ward N. Boylston of Boston. But Thacher checked the facts in William Woodville's *History of the Inoculation of the Small-Pox in Great Britain* (1796) and James Moore's *The History of the Small-Pox* (1815), which told a different story. "Now if your account of Dr Boylston is altogether tradition," he wrote Mr. Boylston gently,

may it not possibly be erroneous? If however you have documents to substantiate the facts, then it must appear as a vile attempt to deprive Dr Boylston of the merit & honor which were justly his due. Should your statement be published & utimately prove erroneous it would excite unpleasant feelings in all concerned. Will you be pleased dear Sir, to take the subject into consideration . . . ?[7]

Mr. Boylston, who was doubtless not accustomed to having his family traditions challenged in this way, did not at first reply. Thacher appealed to a mutual friend, Dr. Shattuck, for help; and Shattuck learned that Mr. Boylston believed the basis of the assertion was a letter from Sir Hans Sloane to Zabdiel Boylston, which, Boylston confessed, was unfortunately "misplaced." The excuse was familiar—and unacceptable. Thacher revised the sketch to conform to the known facts and consigned to a footnote an inoffensively-phrased version of the family tradition, with the reasons for rejecting it.[8]

On the whole Thacher's selections showed sound judgment. He included almost everyone worthy of inclusion and, except for some local New England doctors, few who had neither outstanding achievements nor general reputation. Dr. Hosack thought Thacher ought to have included

[7] Thacher to Boylston, Plymouth, Mass., Nov. 20, 1826, Shattuck Papers, Massachusetts Historical Society.
[8] Thacher to Shattuck, Plymouth, Mass., Dec. 11, 26, 1826, Shattuck Papers.

Hugh Mercer, a military hero as well as a physician; and we may regret, or wonder at, the omission of Peter Fayssoux of Charleston, John Minson Galt of Williamsburg, George Logan of Philadelphia, John Mitchell, the Virginia scientist, and two or three others. To one critic it appeared that the criterion of admission to Thacher's pages was as often civic prominence as medical distinction. In general, however, one cannot seriously quarrel with Thacher's selections. He recognized significant figures like Joshua Clayton of Delaware and Walter Jones of Virginia, even when he was unable to learn much about them. In such cases he told what he knew and said no more—unlike Williams, who began the sketch of one Massachusetts doctor: " I know little or nothing of his early education, but believe it was sufficient to qualify him for entering on the study of the healing art. At least, it was so considered at that early day." [9]

Thacher's *American Medical Biography* has the character and authority of a collection of original sources, for many of Thacher's contributors knew the physicians about whom they wrote and related what they knew in unvarnished prose. Thus we are told that Seth Bird drank to excess, kept his coffin ready at his bedside, and prospered beyond his deserts; and that James Hurlburt ended his days a pauper dependent on his patients' charity, a drunken wreck who would not " even look at a patient till a full bottle was placed in his entire control, and daily replenished." The author of the sketch of Nathan Smith tells us frankly that Smith's operation for the removal of cataracts on Dr. William Aspinwall was unsuccessful, and Aspinwall became blind. Lemuel Hopkins is brought vividly to life in an anecdote: finding the windows of a sick-room tightly closed and curtained, he carried the patient out of doors, stood over her, and fended off the staves and pokers of angry, fearful parents and relations until the child recovered in fresh air. Thacher himself sketched his preceptor Abner Hersey of Barnstaple in all his churlish eccentricity, terrified of smallpox, which he had never had, peevish, rudely inhospitable, uninterested in experiments or the theory of medicine, and at the end bequeathing part of his estate to Harvard College for a chair of anatomy and surgery and the rest to the thirteen churches of Barnstaple County to provide copies of Doddridge's theological works to the parishioners forever.[10]

In addition to such vignettes, Thacher's biographies contain many intriguing references and allusions which ought to stimulate our inquiry.

[9] Williams, *American Medical Biography*, p. 17.
[10] See also Thacher to John Warren, Plymouth, Mass., Jan. 25, 1787, Warren Papers, vol. III, Massachusetts Historical Society.

William Baynham of Virginia, about whom little has been written, is ranked second only to Philip Syng Physick as a surgeon. Richard Bayley of New York, we are told, was better known in France than in his native land. Occasionally a phrase or judgment arrests or amuses us. What were the " untoward events " in Richard Kissam's life? What reservation had Abner Moseley's biographer in mind when he wrote that Moseley's " parents were respectable, especially his mother "? And we know it must be a Yale man who assures us, as Dr. Thomas Miner does in his account of Lemuel Hopkins, that " Connecticut was the seat of the muses in the United States " in the last quarter of the eighteenth century, as though Philadelphia, or even Boston, never existed.

Thacher's book was generally favorably noticed. Dr. Gouverneur Emerson, in the *American Journal of the Medical Sciences,* thought it more interesting than could have been expected, "considering that the lives of physicians, to whatever eminence they may have attained, are seldom distinguished by remarkable adventures or variety of incident." [11] The reviewer in the *Boston Medical and Surgical Journal* found in the book much of interest, and then continued:

The work will in some measure correct the popular notion that physicians are generally sceptical in opinion and relaxed in morals; for it will be seen that a considerable number of the most successful and eminent physicians in this country have been distinguished for their moral and religious character.[12]

Only in New York was the book strongly criticized, and that was because Dr. John B. Beck took exception to Thacher's account of the bitter quarrels in the medical faculty of that city, in which Beck himself had taken part.[13]

Thacher lived fifteen years after the publication of the *American Medical Biography.* During that period he wrote a vigorous exposé of the Salem witchcraft delusion and a solid, carefully researched history of Plymouth, and he took an active part in the affairs of the Pilgrim Society; but he did not continue, as some hoped he would, his medical biographical writing. That was left for Stephen West Williams.

Stephen West Williams (1790-1855)

Son and grandson of physicians of Deerfield, Mass., Williams was born in that attractive village in 1790 and received an education at the

[11] *Am. J. M. Sc.,* 1828, 2: 399-400.

[12] *Boston M. & S. J.,* 1828-29, 1: 223.

[13] *New York M. & Phys. J.,* 1828, 7: 404-416; David Hosack to Thacher, Jan. 1, 1829, Medical College Papers, Rutgers University Archives.

local academy.[14] He studied medicine in his father's office and then spent a year in the medical school of Columbia College, where he was a student of the surgeon Valentine Mott, with whom he remained in friendly correspondence until his death. Returning to Deerfield, Williams soon found that village practice did not challenge his abilities or satisfy his needs. He studied natural history, collected an herbarium, and compiled a record of local plants and flowers, which his wife illustrated with sketches and paintings. By gift and purchase he assembled a collection of books which he boasted was " probably the most extensive of any medical library in this part of the state." [15] From time to time he lectured —at the Berkshire Medical Institution on medical jurisprudence from 1823 to 1831, at the College of Physicians and Surgeons in New York for one winter, at Dartmouth College for two, and at Willoughby University of Lake Erie, Ohio, for two more.

Meanwhile, Williams had begun to write, first on medical and scientific subjects,[16] then on local history. A sketch of the Indians of the Connecticut Valley won him honorary membership in the New-York Historical Society in 1818. From local records and recollections (one of his informants was an ancient dame of 88, " with a memory as elastic as in youth ")[17] Williams compiled the annals of Old Deerfield, and he delivered six public lectures on local history in 1836.[18] Some of this material he incorporated in the notes to a new edition of his ancestor John Williams' account of how he was captured and carried off by the Indians who sacked Deerfield in 1704.[19]

With such background and interests it was natural that Williams should study the medical history of his neighborhood. In 1842 he delivered before the Massachusetts Medical Society an address on the " Medical History of the County of Franklin." [20] He had collected the

[14] For biographical sketches, see *Boston M. & S. J.*, 1855, *53*: 29-32, and New England Historic Genealogical Society, *Memorial Biographies,* vol. II (1881), pp. 389-397.

[15] Williams to George W. Norris, Deerfield, Mass., June 12, 1852, College of Physicians of Philadelphia.

[16] " Floral Calendar kept at Deerfield, Massachusetts, with Miscellaneous Remarks," Jan. 25, 1819, *Am. J. Sc.*, 1818-19, *1*: 359-373; Williams to Hezekiah Howe, Deerfield, Mass., Oct. 1, 1817, Miscellaneous Papers, Manuscript Division, New York Public Library.

[17] " Recollections collected from Mrs. Bradley," ms., Pocomtuck Valley Memorial Association Library, Deerfield.

[18] " Ancient History of Pocomptuck [sic], or Deerfield," ms., Pocomtuck Valley Memorial Association Library.

[19] *A Biographical Memoir of the Rev. John Williams* . . . (Greenfield, Mass., 1837).

[20] " A medical history of the County of Franklin, in the Commonwealth of Massachu-

material for it from the physicians and ministers of the several towns—
bills of mortality, data on births, deaths, climate, and diseases, and
biographical data on famous departed doctors. Like every other historian,
Williams was sometimes frustrated in his research. About Dr. Ebenezer
Barnard (1745-1790) of Deerfield, for example, he could discover almost
nothing, for "his widow, or some of his friends, disposed of his papers,
or deposited them in so obscure a place that I have never been able
to obtain them, much to my regret." [21] The "Medical History of the
County of Franklin" was a workmanlike job, it demonstrated the prob-
able worth of a similar work on a larger scale, and it led directly to
Williams' largest and best remembered work in medical history, his
American Medical Biography.

Williams had ended his account of medicine in Franklin County with
an expression of hope that Thacher would continue his work on American
medical biography. The words were merely a conventional acknowledg-
ment, for Thacher was then 88 years old and Williams had in fact
practically decided to undertake the work himself. He proceeded methodi-
cally. First, he got endorsement of his project from a score of physicians
—from Thacher himself; from the *Boston Medical and Surgical Journal;*
from the venerable Dr. John Redman Coxe and Dr. Isaac Hays, editor
of the *American Journal of the Medical Sciences* in Philadelphia; from
Drs. Mott and John W. Francis in New York; from the historian Col.
William L. Stone of Albany. Samuel B. Wood, superintendent of the
State Mental Hospital at Worcester, Mass., promised help, as did Dr.
Ebenezer Alden of Randolph, who told Williams he had biographical
data, "more or less extensive," on 296 deceased Massachusetts physicians. [22]

Then Williams solicited subscriptions. Dr. Oliver W. Holmes reported
on how he got some at a meeting of the Massachusetts Medical Society:

> I thought the best way would be to introduce the matter at the dinner table
> when I should be called upon, as I expected to be, for a speech or sentiment. I
> therefore took that opportunity to speak of our obligations to our instructors and
> the patriarchs of our art—the debt of gratitude we owe them—our obligation to
> cherish their memory etc. etc. and then after an allusion to the late Dr Thacher

setts," Massachusetts Medical Society, *M. Communications*, 1848, 7: 1-76. See also W.
A. Wilkins to Williams, Leyden, Mass., Dec. 27, 1841, Heritage Foundation, Deerfield,
Mass.

[21] Williams, *American Medical Biography*, p. 30.

[22] *Ibid.*, pp. v-ix; Williams to Jonathan Pereira, April 13, 1843, in "Correspondence
with the late Doctor Jonathan Pereira, of London," *New Jersey M. Reporter*, 1855, 8:
109.

and his work, I turned the current of my remarks to your proposed undertaking, spoke of its interest and value, and sent the subscription paper to the president to be handed about.

It was a great pity that I was not called up earlier, because many of the Society left the room before the paper had a chance to reach them. This however, I could not help—older and wiser men came before me.[23]

Meanwhile Williams had been collecting biographies for the book. True to his word, Dr. Woodward prepared several. Dr. James Jackson of Boston sent a copy of his memoir of his son and a biography of John Gorham (which Williams did not use). From Dr. Francis came a copy of his memoir of David Hosack. Dr. Thomas Sewall of Washington wrote an account of John Godman; while, through the interest of Dr. Isaac Hays, sketches of Philip Syng Physick, Joseph Parrish, Thomas C. James, and others were obtained in Philadelphia. Williams included all but one of the sketches he had written for his Franklin County address, and he transcribed others from the pages of the *Boston Medical and Surgical Journal.* In all 110 biographies were prepared.

Williams' *American Medical Biography,* like Thacher's, presented a cast of interesting characters. Dr. George B. Doane of Boston delivered over 3000 babies in the years between 1820 and 1842, averaging in the last three years of his life not fewer than four a week. Dr. Josiah Goodhue of Putney, Vt., performed an amputation without ever having seen the operation before, and books were his only guides in most of the capital operations he performed. Dr. Pardon Hayes, like other physicians of western Massachusetts, often visited his patients in winter on snowshoes, charging 1*s.* a mile for travel. Dr. Daniel Sheldon took two to four drachms of opium daily for 40 years; he stopped at last in old age, " without detriment," and died in his 90th year. And Caleb Ticknor is characterized as honest, disinterested, and courageous—adjectives not often given to homeopaths in the 1840's.

Not a few of Williams' subjects are described approvingly as " of the old school "—a class of men which, though always dwindling and nearly extinct, appears to survive into every generation. A still larger number are characterized as " facetious," also a term of approval; and a few as robust types who could set a table ringing with laughter. One of these was Dr. Samuel Church (1756-1826) of Sunderland, Mass., who had a famous exchange with Dr. Hunt, also " a man of unbounded humor," who kept a drug store at Northampton. Hunt called on Church in the following terms to pay a bill:

[23] Holmes to Williams, Boston, June 1, 1844, Heritage Foundation.

Dr. Church,
    Dear Sir: I am in want of a fat hog; please send it, or ——
                                                        Ebenezer Hunt

To this Church replied:

Dr. Hunt,
    Dear Sir: I have no fat hog; and if I had ——
                                                        Samuel Church

The *American Medical Biography* appeared in the last weeks of 1844.
It was recognized at once for what Williams intended it—the continuation
of Thacher—and the reviews were generally favorable. The *Boston
Medical and Surgical Journal* declared that as " the whole United States
has been the ground for his [Williams'] inquiries . . . the work possesses
the same intrinsic interest to the reader in New Orleans, or St. Louis,
that it does to us in the city of Boston." [24] But this is precisely the quality
that Williams' book did not have. It could not possibly have appealed
to southern or western physicians as it did to those of New England.
Three quarters of the 110 sketches were of New England or New York
physicians. Only seven names were from Pennsylvania, five from Maryland, three from Virginia, three from Georgia, two from South Carolina,
and one each from New Jersey, the District of Columbia, and Missouri.
The *Medical Examiner* of Philadelphia came closer to the mark when,
in a generally favorable review, it remarked, " We have been surprised,
indeed, to find so many names in the book presented for the first time to
our notice, particularly from Massachusetts and the adjoining states." [25]
    Not only was Williams' work not a national biographical collection,
it had literary deficiencies which affected its usefulness as a collection
of historical sources. Williams had neither written any substantial
number of the biographies nor edited and revised those he took from
other publications. One thinks that Ansel W. Ives (1787-1838), Williams' roommate at Columbia and his " most intimate friend " for many
years, should have been memorialized by Williams himself; instead the
compiler merely reprinted a memoir from the *American Journal of the
Medical Sciences*. In consequence of Williams' editorial carelessness,
there are many irritating confusions. " Died last month " was perfectly
comprehensible in the newspaper or journal in which the obituary first
appeared; the same words, reprinted unchanged by Williams several years
later, are meaningless or misleading.
    Because of these deficiencies and because the book was printed in a

----

[24] *Boston M. & S. J.*, 1845, *32*: 23-24.
[25] *M. Examiner, Philadelphia*, 1845, n. s. *1*: 110-111.

small New England town and had to be promoted by the author un-
assisted, Williams' *American Medical Biography* seems to have had only
a small and slow sale. In Philadelphia, for example, an agent agreed to
take 50 copies on consignment, but at the end of three months he had
disposed of only three.[26]

Williams continued historical study and writing for the remaining
ten years of his life. Two years after the appearance of the *American
Medical Biography*, he published *The Genealogy and History of the
Family of Williams in America* (Greenfield, 1847), for which he collected
material from the Harvard College Library and on personal visits to
members of the family, to some of whom he was directed by Henry
Stevens, the Yankee bookseller in London. By now Williams' reputation
had spread beyond Deerfield. When Francis Parkman visited the village,
Williams was able to show original records, which Parkman later used in
his history of the French and English in North America;[27] and he
assisted Colonel William L. Stone in locating documents for his life of
Sir William Johnson. Samuel G. Drake of the New England Historic
Genealogical Society asked for an article for his journal; but Williams
put him off: "I have many facts from our old town books, & from many
other sources which ought to be published there," Williams explained.
"I wish I had time to prepare them, but I fear I never shall have."[28]

One reason why he could not finish an article for Drake was that he
was preparing his presidential address for the Franklin County Medical
Society. "Notices of some of the medical improvements and discoveries
of the last half century" was his most thoughtful historical work.[29] As
he had done when preparing his earlier books and articles, Williams
sought help in this; but as he was treating a broad subject, he solicited
data beyond the circle of Massachusetts antiquaries. For example, he
asked Valentine Mott for a sketch of the progress of surgery in the
preceding fifty years; but Mott declined, on the ground that he would
have to state too often that the improvements had been his.[30]

In this presidential address Williams spoke not only of medical discoveries—one of the most beneficent improvements he thought was the

[26] G. B. Zieber & Co. to Williams, Philadelphia, Jan. 24, April 13, 1846, Heritage
Foundation.

[27] Williams to Parkman, Deerfield, Mass., Nov. 15, 1851, Parkman Papers, Massachusetts Historical Society.

[28] Williams to Drake, Deerfield, Mass., July 21, 1851, Dreer Collection, Historical
Society of Pennsylvania.

[29] *New York J. Med.*, 1852, n. s. *8*: 153-186.

[30] Mott to Williams, New York, April 5, 1851, Heritage Foundation.

more moderate use of drugs—but of the improvements of medical education on every level. The average eighteenth-century medical library contained between 25 and 150 volumes—the works of Cullen, Brown, Sydenham, Willis, Pringle, Darwin's *Zoonomia,* with Boerhaave, Van Swieten, and Fothergill, represented in only a few libraries. Some doctors, in fact, had not so many: Williams related with a note of incredulity that Dr. Dexter of Topsfield, who died in 1783, was a popular and successful physician though he owned " just two books." By the middle of the nineteenth century all this was changing. No doctor's library could be very useful or be thought complete which did not contain several medical journals. " I consider good medical journals the best possible books for all times, which can be or are published . . . they are books for the ages." A physician in 1850 could no more practice without books and journals, Williams went on, than a mechanic could work without tools; and those who decried books and pretended to practice on experience only he dismissed as " modern wiseacres."

Williams had made several visits to the West. In the summer of 1851 he travelled in the upper Mississippi Valley, which " highly delighted " him. He inspected Indian mounds; at Detroit he " pondered over " the history of Pontiac's war; and throughout he kept a journal, which he thought of publishing.[31] Two years later, in 1853, in poor health, he left Deerfield, with all its personal and ancestral ties, to live at Laona in northern Illinois with his son Edward Jenner Williams. Here, as at Deerfield, he interested himself in local history and in 1855 was invited to deliver the annual Fourth of July address.[32] He prepared it carefully, but it is doubtful that he read it, for he became ill on July 2 and died one week later.

Samuel David Gross (1805-1884)

Ten years after the publication of Williams' biographical dictionary, Samuel D. Gross, surgeon and teacher in Louisville, Ky., issued a prospectus for yet another American medical biography. Gross was by far an abler and more famous member of the medical profession than either Thacher or Williams, and his medical biography reflected his broader vision, careful planning, and vigorous editorial control.

Samuel D. Gross was born in 1805 on a farm near Easton, Pa., where

---

[31] He wrote " A Complete History of Mount Auburn, Ohio," 1843, the ms. of which is in Yale University Library.

[32] Williams, " American Independence," Laona, Ill., July 4, 1855, ms., Pocomtuck Valley Memorial Association Library.

he sometimes amused himself and entertained his playmates by killing woodpeckers by means of an ingenious device that caused a concussion of their nervous systems.[33] He had an uncertain elementary education, largely in German, in local country schools, but overcame the deficiencies by attending academies in Wilkes-Barre, New York, and Lawrenceville before commencing the study of medicine and entering Jefferson Medical College in Philadelphia. After several years' practice in Philadelphia, where he began to translate and write on surgical subjects, he moved to Ohio, where he taught at the Cincinnati Medical College for five years and at the University of Louisville for sixteen. By 1856, when he was appointed to the professorship of surgery at Jefferson, he had achieved wide reputation as a practitioner, teacher, and writer and had begun to prepare his *System of Surgery,* one of the greatest works in the field. A tireless worker, he once explained his prodigious output as the consequence of his habit of working systematically while other men slept, smoked cigars, lounged about their houses, or spent their evenings in entertainments.[34]

Gross had always been, as he said, "passionately fond of books," called them his "friends," and owned more than 5000 volumes when he died, including a large collection of "the Fathers of Surgery." He liked to recall that he had bought heavily at the sale of John Redman Coxe's library, leaving an unlimited bid for Paracelsus' *Opera Omnia* (Geneva, 1658). He got the volumes for $54 but, on learning that Coxe's grandson was the underbidder, offered them to him. Five years later, on the younger man's death, the books were put up once more, and Gross bought them for $7.[35] Sometimes Gross longed for leisure to study these old volumes, compare their doctrines and practice, and write commentaries on them. If such notes were accompanied by biographical sketches, he thought, they would be more valuable. "I am not one of those who believe that our ancestors were fools," he wrote.[36]

Gross' first opportunity to prepare a biographical essay came in 1852 when he was called on for a memorial address on Daniel Drake. In the six weeks he had to prepare it, he collected a vast amount of information, made use of Drake's "Reminiscential Letters to his Children," and

---

[33] Samuel D. Gross, *Autobiography* (2 vols., Philadelphia, 1887), *passim.*

[34] Gross, *History of American Medical Literature, from 1776 to the Present Time* (Philadelphia, 1876).

[35] Gross, *Autobiography,* vol. II, pp. 8-10. The volumes are now in the Gross Library in the College of Physicians of Philadelphia, as Dr. W. B. McDaniel II has determined for me.

[36] *Ibid.,* p. 10.

American Medical Biography.

The undersigned proposes to publish, within the next twelve months, a work entitled "Memoirs of Distinguished American Physicians and Surgeons," to be comprised in two duodecimo volumes of about 400 pages each. In order to insure greater excellence, each Biography will be furnished by a separate contributor; and as the work is intended for popular use, it is desirable that it should be as free as possible from technicalities. The work will be put to press on the first of September next, and the proceeds, if any, will be distributed, *pro rata*, among the different contributors. Each sketch must not be less than fifteen pages, nor more than thirty-five. The Memoirs will comprise the folllowing names, with, perhaps, a few others:

BARD, SAMUEL	LUZENBERG, C. A.
BARTLETT, ELISHA	McCLELLAN, GEORGE
BARTON, B. S.	McDOWELL, EPHRAIM
BEAUMONT, WILLIAM	McNEVEN, W. J.
BECK, J. B.	MILLER, EDWARD
BECK, T. R.	MITCHELL, S. L.
CALDWELL, CHARLES	MORTON, S. G.
CHAPMAN, N.	PARRISH, JOSEPH
COOKE, J. E.	
DANA, J. F.	PHYSICK, P. S.
DAVIDGE, J. B.	POST, WRIGHT
DEWEES, W. P.	RAMSAY, DAVID
DORSEY, J. S.	RANDOLPH, JACOB
DRAKE, DANIEL	REVERE, JOHN
EBERLE, JOHN	RODGERS, J. K.
GODMAN, J. D.	ROGERS, J. B.
HARTSHORNE, JOSEPH	RUSH, BENJAMIN
HOLYOKE, E. A.	SHIPPEN, WILLIAM
HARRISON, J. P.	SMITH, NATHAN
HOSACK, DAVID	SWETT, JOHN
HORNER, W. E.	THATCHER, JAMES
JACKSON, JAMES, Jr.,	WARREN, JOHN
JAMES, T. C.	WELLS, J. D.
JONES, JOHN	WISTAR CASPAR

From the above list it will be seen that the work will comprise none but the names of those who have earned a national reputation. The only motive which the Editor has in superintending its publication is his desire to popularize his profession, and to place its services more conspicuously than has yet been done before the American people.

S. D. GROSS.

Louisville, Dec. 10, 1855.

Fig. 2. Gross' 1855 prospectus. Courtesy of the College of Physicians of Philadelphia

endeavored to make the address inspiring as well as instructive.[37] Though some thought it too long—a friend said that in his biographical writings as distinguished from his scientific articles Gross did " not possess the art of leaving things unsaid " [38]—the general effect was good. One result of this exercise was that Gross conceived the scheme of preparing an American medical biography " for popular use." He may also have been stimulated to this when he realized that, with the deaths of Nathaniel Chapman and William E. Horner within a year of Drake's, an era in American medicine was closing and should be recorded. The prospectus, issued in 1855, contained the names of forty-eight subjects, all men of national reputation; each sketch would run from fifteen to thirty-five pages, making two volumes duodecimo of 400 pages each; and the work was to be completed within the twelve-month.[39]

For some subjects—among them Benjamin Smith Barton, William Beaumont, Charles Caldwell, Edward A. Holyoke, John Jones, Edward Miller, Wright Post, David Ramsay, William Shippen, Jr., and Nathan Smith—Gross could not find an author; while some potential authors declined his invitations and resisted his importunities. To George W. Norris of Philadelphia, author of an excellent, but then still unpublished, " Early History of Medicine in Philadelphia," Gross wrote:

I must have a Memoir of Dr. Physick, worthy of the man, the profession, & the country. You knew Physick personally, you are a surgeon, & you are one of his *immediate* fellow-citizens. I, therefore, appeal to you to furnish me with a suitable sketch of the life of that illustrious man for my contemplated work. Write 30, 40, or 50 pages, as you please. It will be in time if your MS. reaches me by the 1st of September. I shall take no refusal. You, of all men, are *the* man to serve me in this respect. The subject is worthy of your pen & talents.[40]

Norris was unmoved by the appeal, and Gross was no more successful in getting from him a revision of his published memoir of Jacob Randolph.[41] The sketch of Physick was done by Dr. John Bell of Philadelphia, who asked $100 for it.[42]

The appearance of *Lives of Eminent American Physicians and Surgeons of the Nineteenth Century* was delayed three or four years by

---

[37] *A Discourse on the Life, Character, and Services of Daniel Drake, M. D.* (Louisville, 1853).

[38] J. M. DaCosta, " Biographical sketch of Professor Samuel D. Gross," American Philosophical Society, *Proceedings*, vol. XXII (1885), p. 82.

[39] Gross, " American Medical Biography," Louisville, Dec. 10, 1855 (handbill), College of Physicians of Philadelphia.

[40] Gross to Norris, Louisville, May 17, 1856, College of Physicians of Philadelphia.

[41] Gross to Norris, Louisville, June 13, 1856, College of Physicians of Philadelphia.

[42] Gross, *Autobiography*, vol. I, p. 143.

the Panic of 1857; it appeared at last early in 1861. The biographies were arranged in chronological order, beginning with Benjamin Rush, so that they formed a sort of consecutive account of the development of medicine in America. Of the thirty-two sketches, twenty-six had been in Gross' prospectus, and six—those of Samuel Brown, Amariah Brigham, Lewis C. Beck, Charles Frick, Moreton Stillé, and John Collins Warren —were new. The selection could not be criticized for parochial bias—all thirty-two were persons of distinction, even of national reputation. Every sketch was long enough—Physick's ran to 109 pages—to allow each author to discuss his subject in some detail, with ample references to sources. Gross himself contributed three—on John Syng Dorsey, Daniel Drake, and Ephraim McDowell. The life of Dorsey was enriched with quotations from Dorsey's letters from London and Paris, where he had studied; while the sketch of McDowell contains a scholarly examination of the basis of that surgeon's fame and a sympathetic account of his career and character. If Gross' *Lives* recorded none of the quirkiness so abundant in Thacher's sketches of Yankee doctors, they are more valuable for their critical judgments. Gross gave several pages to a description of McDowell's operation, while the biography of Charles Frick is almost entirely an account of work in urological surgery.

Unfortunately Gross' book appeared just as the Civil War broke, when attention was drawn elsewhere. The sale was consequently poor, and Gross' keenest memory of the work seemed to be that it cost him $200 of his own money, with no compensating royalties.[43]

Though a financial failure, the *Lives* established Gross' reputation as a medical biographer and historian. The mere passage of time added to his fame, for Gross lived long enough to become himself a historical figure, with his personal memories the stuff of history. He wrote other biographical memoirs of deceased friends and colleagues, like Charles Wilkins Short, Valentine Mott, Robley Dunglison, Isaac Hays, and J. Marion Sims, and published a biographical account of Ambroise Paré[44] and a book on John Hunter and his pupils. For public lectures at Jefferson Medical College he sometimes chose historical themes, as in 1867, when he gave a thoughtful, stimulating, often entertaining recital of changes and progress in medicine in his lifetime, and in 1871, when he presented a series of vignettes of his Jefferson teachers George and Samuel McClellan, John Eberle, Jacob Green, William P. C. Barton, and

[43] *Ibid.*

[44] " A sketch of the life, character, and services of Ambroise Paré," *North Am. Med.-Chir. Rev.*, 1861, 5: 1059-1083. Gross delivered the same address before the Jefferson students, Feb. 12, 1873, when it was published separately.

B. Rush Rhees.[45] For the American Medical Association he had prepared in 1856 a thoughtful " Report on the Causes which Impede the Progress of American Medical Literature ";[46] twenty years later he issued a kind of sequel, two lectures later issued in book form as *The History of American Medical Literature, from 1776 to the Present Time,* which recorded the striking advances of a generation and expressed his confidence in the future development of medical science in America. His autobiography, full of illuminating portraits of his contemporaries, both medical and lay, was Gross' last contribution to the history of his beloved profession.[47]

The biographical dictionaries of Thacher, Williams, and Gross are, of course, valuable for the facts and near-facts they contain about a good many American physicians and surgeons. In not a few instances, these are the only sketches we have; in many, as a comparison with Kelly and Burrage's *American Medical Biography* clearly shows, they are the principal sources from which other, more accessible sketches have been drawn. Most scholars have used these three works—when they have used them at all—as dictionaries are generally used—to search for particular facts about a particular person. Few have read them through, as one reads a history. That is an exercise warmly to be recommended to all historians of medicine in America.

For from reading these nineteenth-century medical biographical dictionaries the historian will make the acquaintance of a number of men who were significant in their own time and are at least interesting in ours— Jason Valentine O'Brien Lawrence, practitioner and teacher of medicine in Philadelphia; Hugh Williamson, whose remarkable career reminds one at once of his contemporary Rush's achievements; the Rev. Matthew Wilson of Lewes, Del., a cleric physician who wrote about climate and diseases; William P. Dewees, the able and appealing professor of midwifery at the University of Pennsylvania; and Valentine Seaman, one of the early vaccinators. Only a handful of the men whom Thacher, Williams, and Gross included in their books have ever been subjects of modern biographical treatment on any scale and of whatever quality. Most do not seem to deserve such neglect. One ventures therefore to propose that historians and biographers should declare a moratorium on

[45] *Then and Now: A Discourse Introductory to the Forty-third Course of Lectures in the Jefferson Medical College of Philadelphia* (Philadelphia, 1867) ; *An Address Delivered before the Alumni Association of the Jefferson Medical College . . . 1871* (Philadelphia, 1871).

[46] American Medical Association, *Transactions,* vol. IX (1856), pp. 339-362.

[47] Gross, *Autobiography,* vol. II, pp. 236 ff.

research and writing about Rush, Osler, and a few others, and turn their attention instead to men like John Eberle, Edward Cutbush, Edward Miller, William J. Macneven, and Henry Stuber. Why should not someone complete Gross' original plan by editing a volume of biographies of the twenty-two physicians whom he originally proposed for his *Lives* but did not finally include in it?

More than this, the historian who reads these biographical volumes through from cover to cover will get a picture of medical practice and professional life not readily obtainable otherwise. Here, the local loyalties of Thacher and Williams are actually an advantage to the historian. A good deal is known about the practice of the eminent physicians of Philadelphia, Boston, and New York; the sketches of Thacher's and William's forgotten country doctors provide a clearer idea of what sort of physician served the majority of Americans, at least in the eastern states in the century between 1750 and 1850.

The picture of medicine that will emerge from the pages of these medical biographical dictionaries may very well contain facts or ideas which will cause the historian to sharpen or reconsider the accepted generalizations of American medical history. The practice of medicine and surgery, we know, was usually combined in one person in rural America, as it was once throughout America and is still in much of the United States to this day. What then are we to make of Thomas Hubbard's experience at Pomfret, Conn., early in the nineteenth century? Williams tells us that Hubbard encountered opposition when he sought to combine medicine to surgery, that his justification of the practice on economic grounds fell on deaf ears?[48] Was Williams misinformed? Was Pomfret an unexplained variation from the national norm? Did communities accept the notion of a physician performing the manual operations of surgery, but oppose a surgeon's presuming to practice medicine? Or should the generalization about the union of medicine and surgery be reexamined?

The reading of Thacher, Williams, and Gross offers still another reward to the historian, more personal and subjective, but nonetheless real. He is sure to delight in the cranky plainness of Thacher's style, admire the sweep of judgment of Gross' collaborators, and, above all, have a sense of participating with Thacher, Williams, and Gross in laying foundations for not a little of the writing that has been done in the past century on the history of medicine in the United States.

[48] Williams, *American Medical Biography*, pp. 294-295.

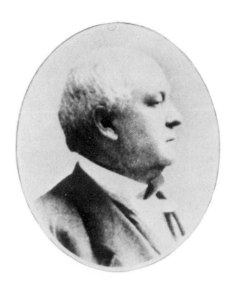

JOSEPH M. TONER

JOSEPH M. TONER (1825-1896) AS A MEDICAL HISTORIAN *

Medical historiography in America has a long tradition. As early as 1769 Peter Middleton of New York, in an introductory lecture, presented a long, discursive account of the development of medicine from ancient times to his own day; and 35 years later, drawing on the experience of half a century, Benjamin Rush recalled for his students the conditions of medical practice in Philadelphia when he was an apprentice in 1760. Growing national consciousness and pride, expressed during the semi-centennial of American independence, doubtless provided strong motives to investigate the history of medicine, as they did the history of other aspects of American life. In 1828 James Thacher of Plymouth, Mass., who had already published the journal of his experiences as a surgeon in the Revolutionary War, compiled an *American Medical Biography*. John B. Beck of Albany wrote a short history of medicine in the colonies for the New York State Medical Society, which was expanded and published in 1850. There were local histories, too, like Ebenezer Allen's on the medical profession of Norfolk County, Massachusetts; while occasionally, on some anniversary, an elderly

* Presidential address delivered at the 45th annual meeting of the American Association for the History of Medicine, Montreal, Canada, May 5, 1972.

practitioner might describe men and events of bygone days, as Jeremiah Spofford did every ten years between 1840 and 1870 to the Essex North District Medical Society in Massachusetts. Samuel D. Gross' scholarly *Lives of Eminent American Physicians and Surgeons of the Nineteenth Century,* published in 1861, rounded out the century that opened with the founding of the first American medical school in 1765.[1]

The quarter century after 1865 witnessed both a notable increase in the amount of historical writing about American medicine, and also a striking improvement in its quality, for authors now chose broader themes and employed printed and manuscript sources more assiduously than their predecessors. Joseph Carson's *History of the Medical Department of the University of Pennsylvania* appeared in 1866. Oliver Wendell Holmes' Massachusetts Historical Society lecture on "The Medical Profession in Massachusetts" was delivered in 1869 (although he had employed history to good advantage 25 years before in "Homeopathy and its Kindred Delusions").[2] Permanently useful one-volume histories of medicine in New Jersey by Stephen W. Wickes appeared in 1879;[3] in Massachusetts by Samuel A. Green in 1881; in Baltimore by John R. Quinan in 1884; in early Philadelphia by George W. Norris in 1886. A biography of John Warren was published in 1873. From the list of its medical graduates which Edinburgh University published in 1867, Samuel Lewis of Philadelphia, himself an Edinburgh graduate, compiled in 1888 the names of American students.[4]

[1] W. B. McDaniel, 2d, "The beginnings of American medical historiography," *Bull. Hist. Med.,* 1952, *26*: 45-53; Whitfield J. Bell, Jr., "Lives in medicine: the biographical dictionaries of Thacher, Williams, and Gross," *ibid.,* 1968, *42*: 101-20; Benjamin Rush, "An inquiry into the comparative state of medicine, in Philadelphia, between the years 1760 and 1766, and the year 1805," *Medical Inquiries* (2nd ed., Philadelphia, 1805), IV, 365-405; John B. Beck, *An Historical Sketch of the State of Medicine in the American Colonies* (Albany, N. Y., 1850, reprinted with foreword by Charles F. Fishback, Albuquerque, N. M., 1966); Ebenezer Alden, "Early history of the medical profession in Norfolk Co.," *Boston Med. & Surg. J.,* 1853, *49*: 149-56, 173-79, 199-205, 215-20, 237-40, and separately; Jeremiah Spofford to Toner, Jan. 1, 1875, Toner Papers, No. 91 (Manuscript Division, Library of Congress). Spofford, who was well into his 80s when he wrote Toner, remembered Edward Holyoke, John Warren, William Eustis, James Thacher, and others of the Revolutionary generation.

[2] Holmes' lectures on homeopathy, 1842, and on medicine in Massachusetts, 1869, may be found in his *Medical Essays,* in the Riverside edition of his collected *Writings,* IX. See also his "Additional Memoranda" to Samuel A. Green's chapter on "Medicine in Boston" in Justin Winsor, ed., *Memorial History of Boston* (Boston, 1883), IV, 549-70.

[3] In 1875 Wickes edited and published *Minutes and Proceedings of the New Jersey Medical Society, 1776-1800;* the remaining minutes to 1858 appeared in 1881.

[4] Samuel Lewis, "List of the American graduates in medicine in the University

One of those who encouraged, and in his career illustrated, this quickening interest in medical history was Joseph Meredith Toner, a practicing physician of Washington, D. C., a leader in the profession who became president of both the American Medical Association and the American Public Health Association, a scholarly man with a taste for literary and antiquarian pursuits. As the author of historical monographs, the collector of a large library, and the promoter of commemorative events, he made important contributions to the history of medicine in the generation preceding that dominated by Mitchell and Osler.[5]

Born in Pittsburgh in 1825 of an Irish Catholic family settled in Pennsylvania for several generations, Toner grew up on a farm, was apprenticed at 17 to a carriage-builder and wagon-maker, attended the Western University of Pennsylvania for a year and Mount St. Mary's College at Emmitsburg, Md., for two. He tried several jobs—bought and operated a canal boat, clerked in a store—but finally in 1847, at the age of 22, began to study medicine with Dr. John Lowman of Johnstown, Pa. During the winter of 1849-50 he and Lowman attended classes at Jefferson Medical College in Philadelphia. In his diary young Toner noted that Robley Dunglison lectured a whole hour " without ever stopping to take breath, " that Charles D. Meigs one morning delivered " a flaming lecture on dynamics of labor " which " had the whole class in roars of laughter several times, " and that a patient who had been operated under " chloria eather " for removal of a tumor from his thigh, announced on regaining consciousness that " he had just been having the pleasantest dream that ever he had in his life. "[6] When the Jefferson term closed, Toner went to Woodstock, Vt., where three months later, in June 1850, he received an M. D. degree from the Vermont College of Medicine, presenting a thesis on the surgical method of arresting hemorrhage. For a time Toner practiced at Summit, Pa., a village of 200-300 on the Allegheny Portage Railroad; but in the winter of 1852-53

of Edinburgh, " *New England Historical and Genealogical Register,* 1888, *42*: 159-65.

[5] The principal biographical sketches are by Ainsworth R. Spofford in Philosophical Society of Washington, *Bulletin,* 1895-99, *13*: 426-30, and in Smithsonian Institution, *Annual Report, 1896* (Washington, 1898), 637-43; by Thomas Antisell in Toner, *Address before the Rocky Mountain Medical Association, June 6, 1877* (Washington, 1877), 388-405; by Martin F. Morris, " Memorial of Joseph Meredith Toner, " Columbia Historical Society, *Records,* 1897, *1*: 177-84; and memorial addresses in Medical Society of the District of Columbia, *Transactions,* n. s., 1897, *1*: 135-58.

[6] Toner, Diary, Jan. 4, 30, 1850, Toner Papers, No. 60.

he returned to Jefferson, where he received a second doctor's degree in 1853.

For the next two years Toner practiced, first at Pittsburgh, then at Harper's Ferry, Va. Neither place was congenial. He thought of settling in Louisville, Ky., where he was assured the large Roman Catholic population offered the prospect of good practice and income; he offered his services to the Russian minister as a military surgeon in the Crimea; and he was eager to serve in the severe yellow fever epidemic in Norfolk, Va., in 1855. Finally, in the fall of that year, he moved to Washington, and there he remained for the rest of his life.[7]

In Washington Toner quickly associated himself with the Catholic community, joined in founding Catholic hospitals and orphanages, which he then served as attending physician. Though unmarried—there is evidence that he was in love with a young lady of Summit, who entered a convent in 1851[8]—he did not join the Union Army, but remained in Washington, where, as a civilian, he attended the sick and wounded in the military hospitals. Toner's reputation was soon established beyond the Catholic community—the Smithsonian Institution summoned him to attend George Catlin during the last months of the artist's life.[9] His practice grew and his investments prospered; by 1865 he was in comfortable circumstances, with a wide circle of friends and sufficient leisure for his avocations.

Toner was an active member of the Medical Society of the District of Columbia; he was chairman of its library committee, a determined promoter of plans for a permanent hall, and finally its president. He began to attend the annual meetings of the American Medical Association, was named in 1868 to the committee to consider the practicability of the Association's establishing a library (which was done the next year),[10]

[7] Charles J. Boeswald to Toner, Jan. 6, 1855; William Walsh to Toner, Nov. 1, 1855, ibid., No. 2; "Biographical Sketch of J. M. Toner, M. D.," Northwestern Med. & Surg. J., 1873, 3: 247-50.

[8] Ginnie Josephine Warde to Toner, Aug. 10, 1851, Toner Papers, No. 2.

[9] William J. Rhees to Toner, Oct. 4, 1872, ibid., No. 9.

[10] The history of this library is related by Marjorie H. Moore in Morris Fishbein, A History of the American Medical Association, 1847 to 1947 (Philadelphia: Saunders, 1947), 1071-78. Toner's correspondence shows that he took a major part: he drafted the committee's report, which, adopted by the Association, was the library's charter; he circularized a printed appeal to the members of the Association for books; and he made arrangements, first with the Medical Society of the District of Columbia and the Library of Congress, then with the Secretary of the Smithsonian Institution, for the deposit of the books. A. R. Spofford to Toner, April 3, 1869; Joseph Henry to Toner, April 28, 1870; Nathan S. Davis to Toner, Dec. 3, 1868, Sept. 22, 1869;

and in 1873 was elected president. In his presidential address Toner pointed out the importance of laboratory and other modern technical methods in the diagnosis and treatment of disease, and urged his professional colleagues to take firm positions of leadership in promoting public health measures.[11]

Public health in fact received more of Toner's attention than medical science. In the American Public Health Association, of which he was also president, Toner called for an extension of what he called state medicine, for more boards of health and better laws, for preventive health measures, and for the conservation of natural resources. Pure drinking water, he asserted at one point, is essential for the health of the people; streams should everywhere be protected from pollution. " Every housekeeper within a city corporation," he continued, "is entitled to an adequate amount of pure potable water. *A manufacturing establishment, however, has no such right.*"[12]

Many of Toner's professional writings were on aspects of public health; most employed statistics in some way. Appreciating the relation of physical elevation to health and disease, Toner prepared, largely from historical records, a list of North American cities and towns where yellow fever and malaria had occurred, and where, considering elevations, temperatures and rainfall, the diseases might be expected to break out again.[13] Fully aware that the summer months were a time of disease and suffering for the poor in urban areas, he proposed that parks be established where mothers might take their "sick and debilitated children " during the summer months to enjoy fresh air, clean water and milk, fresh fruits and vegetables, in hygienic surroundings.[14] Citing

Charles A. Lee to Toner, Aug. 19, 1869, Toner Papers, Nos. 7, 8, 73, 84. Though warmly approved in principle, the National Medical Library was neither supported nor used by the American Medical Association or by practicing physicians. It did not grow, was soon overshadowed by the Surgeon-General's Library, and in 1894 the Association authorized its removal to the Newberry Library in Chicago. In 1907 the Newberry sent it to the John Crerar Library in the same city.

[11] Fishbein, *History of the American Medical Association*, 87-89.

[12] Toner, *An Address on some of the leading Public Health Questions* (American Public Health Association, Public Health Papers, II, 1875), 8.

[13] Toner, " The natural history and geographical limits of yellow fever within the United States," reprinted from *Charleston Med. J. & Rev.,* n. s., 1874, *2,* in *Contributions to the Study of Yellow Fever* (Washington, 1874), 3-36.

[14] Toner, "Free parks and camping grounds; or sanitariums for the sick and debilitated children of large cities, during the summer months," *Northwestern Med. & Surg. J.* 1872, *3:* 167-75. This paper was expanded in *The Sanitarian,* 1873, *1:* 71-81. " The State," wrote Toner, "has a direct moral and pecuniary interest in the health and lives of her citizens." *Ibid.,* 72.

his tables, he predicted that people would soon prefer the mountains to the seashore for vacations, and surmised "that there may be found a region in some part of New Mexico, perhaps as favorable for patients suffering from Phthsis, as can be found within the boundaries of the United States. "[15]

Toner appears to have come to history from the study of public health and medicine. While preparing in 1864 an argument for compulsory vaccination against smallpox, he became interested in the early history of inoculation, and turned aside to write papers on the subject in Massachusetts and Pennsylvania. The latter was an excellent survey of inoculation in that state from the beginning to the introduction of vaccination by John Redman Coxe in 1802. It contained a good deal of general Philadelphia medical history and biography, much of it gleaned from newspapers, and included in a long footnote an account of Dr. Lauchlin Maclean, for whom it was claimed he was the author of *Letters of Junius*.[16]

In 1866 Toner was invited to speak at the anniversary meeting of the Medical Society of the District of Columbia. He chose to tell the story of the Society, which was also much of the story of medicine in Washington. The resulting monograph foreshadowed much of Toner's future work as a medical historian; in method and content it was one of his best; and it established his reputation as the best informed person in the city on historical subjects.[17]

The Medical Society was founded in 1817, although Washington physicians had met occasionally for specific purposes before that date. For many years the Society's progress was uncertain, for it was weakened by internal dissensions, regarded with suspicion by the public and the Congress, and its strength drawn off by rival organizations. No minutes or other systematic records of its early years survived; even the date of founding was in doubt. Toner had therefore to reconstruct its history

[15] Toner, *Annual Oration before the Medical and Chirurgical Faculty of Maryland, April 14, 1875. Contribution to the Medical History and Physical Geography of Maryland* (Baltimore, 1875), 30; *Dictionary of Elevations and Climatic Register of the United States* (New York, 1874), xxii.

[16] Toner, "A paper on the propriety and necessity of compulsory vaccination," American Medical Association, *Transactions*, 1865, *16*: 307-30; "Inoculation in Pennsylvania," Medical Society of the State of Pennsylvania, *Transactions*, 4th ser., pt. 1 (1865), 163-82; "History of inoculation in Massachusetts," Massachusetts Medical Society, *Journal*, 1867, *2*: 151-204.

[17] Toner, *Anniversary Oration delivered before the Medical Society of the District of Columbia, September 26, 1866* (Washington, 1869).

from its charter, miscellaneous manuscripts and printed forms and books, and notices in the *National Intelligencer.* As he pored over the pages of Washington newspapers for references to the Society, Toner's view broadened, for he found many data on the profession as a whole. The printed address contained brief accounts of the medical schools and hospitals of the District, a list of all the 71 buildings that housed sick and wounded soldiers during the Civil War, tables of the ratio of physicians to the general population in successive decades, and a bibliography of the writings of Washington physicians, most of which, Toner remarked, " are in my possession. "

Newspapers, Toner now realized, were an important source, mostly untapped, of information about the medical profession and medical practice, indeed about many aspects of social history. Accordingly, Toner engaged a young woman to winnow the data from the file of the *Pennsylvania Gazette* in the Library Company of Philadelphia, and make an index slip for every report of health, disease, medicine, doctors, and, Toner reminded her, " advertisements of even quack Doctors." [18] The notes thus made were assembled alphabetically and mounted in a large scrapbook : [19]

Abcess of the lung—a case of Dr. DeNormandie. 19 Dec. 1771
C A of New Jersey— a paper on preparation for inoculation and a review of Heberden's paper. 21 June 1760
Ague—specific pill for cure of. 20 Aug. 1783

The *Pennsylvania Gazette* index proved so useful that Toner compiled other indexes—of all the physicians mentioned in Thacher's *Military Journal* and *American Medical Biography,* for example. Good indexes, it was clear, were the key to historical sources of all kinds, and he made them with unflagging industry and enthusiasm. He also prepared an index of the names of persons and places mentioned in Bishop Meade's *Old Churches, Ministers and Families of Virginia,* and a subject index of the contents of all American medical journals. [20]

[18]Toner to Miss L. Pierce, March 10, 1869, Toner Papers, No. 1 ; Fanny M. Leahey to Toner, Nov. 3, 1866, *ibid.,* No. 6.

[19] " Index to Medical Matters found in the Pennsylvania Gazette from its first Issue to the close of 1800, " Toner Papers, No. 170.

[20] Toner, " Index to Names of Persons and Churches in Bishop Meade's Old Churches, Ministers and Families of Virginia," revised by Hugh A. Morrison in Southern History Association, *Publications,* XI, No. 4, supplement (1898). Toner failed to interest a publisher in his index to medical journals. Henry C. Lea to Toner, Jan. 23, 1871, Toner Papers, No. 8.

By 1865 Toner had determined to undertake a biographical dictionary of American physicians. He explained his purpose and requirements in a printed questionnaire and circular.[21]

Hundreds of physicians [the circular read] have died in different parts of the United States, after devoting a long and useful life to their profession, of whose existence and labors there is no record. This should not be so. The want of a work furnishing an outline of the lives of American physicians has long been felt; and that the project meets the approbation of the profession and of the relatives of the deceased medical men, has already been evinced by valuable contributions from different parts of the country.

The questionnaire introduced by this announcement contained 21 queries, mostly asking for specific details of birth, parentage, education, places of residence, and publications, but ending with a stern injunction.

XX. Any particulars not coming within the above—property accumulated, personal appearance, copy of or reference to any biographical sketch, or obituary notice, in professional or popular prints. Engraving and autograph desired, and, if obtainable, any specimens of writing, published or unpublished. If there be any likeness, mention the artist and possessor. Omit nothing which will give interest to a biographical sketch.

Toner sent the circular to other physicians, to children and grand-children of physicians, to postmasters, newspaper editors, and local historians; to anyone who might be able to help in his quest for data on America's deceased physicians. Medical journals printed Toner's appeal, and he himself continued to mail out copies for many years. Though the questionnaire required detailed knowledge and research to answer, to an astonishing extent the recipients were disposed to help. " Dr. Hough handed me one of your circulars soliciting data for Sketches of Deceased American Physicians," wrote the proprietor of the Livingston Republican Power Press Printing Establishment of Geneseo, N. Y.[22]

I called in Dr. Lauderdale of this village, who has long been an officer of the County Med. Society, who sat down with me and we counted up seventeen physicians who had died in this county and of whom we may secure the necessary data. The County medical society is soon to meet in this village. If you will send me the necessary blanks I will see to it that the matter is attended to. Your enterprise is most praise-worthy.

Others were equally forthcoming. Dr. George Bacon Wood of Phila-

[21] The printed "Circular Soliciting Information for a Biographical Dictionary of Deceased American Physicians" and early ms. drafts are in Toner Papers, No. 64.
[22] L. L. Doty to Toner, May 3, 1870, ibid., No. 8.

delphia sent Toner copies of his obituary memoirs of Joseph Parrish, Samuel G. Morton, and Franklin Bache, and a catalogue of medical graduates of the University of Pennsylvania.[23] Some persons, in addition to providing biographical data, suggested the names of others who could help, and names of physicians for inclusion in the biographical dictionary.[24] Only one or two demurred at the prospect of a complete biographical sketch of the recently dead. " Many eminent physicians here—I regret to say it," explained Dr. O. D. Palmer of Beaver County, Pa.,[25]

died by intemperate habits. If we observe the Latin maxim, *De mortuis nil nisi bonum,* we cannot give the true cause of the decease; if we substitute *verum* for *bonum,* friends will complain. I have especially in view two or three German Colleagues. This class of practitioners is strongly represented in Pennsylvania, and many of them popular and successful. Many of these have been educated for surgeons, in Germany, a profession much *below* that of *Doctor....*

Within three or four years Toner had collected biographical notes on 4,000 American physicians, and expected that his file would have " when completed 10,000 which will give it a national character." [26] The first publication to come from Toner's questionnaire was *Contributions to the Annals of Medical Progress and Medical Education in the United States before and during the War of Independence,* which he compiled at the request of the Convention of School Superintendents in Washington in 1872 and which was published by the Government Printing Office in 1874. Neither methodical nor exhaustive, uneven in the treatment of related or parallel topics, the *Contributions* nonetheless furnished a mass of historical and biographical information, much of it collected and published for the first time, for a history of medicine and the profession in the United States. Toner himself regarded the book " rather as memoranda for the use of those interested in similar studies, than as an attempt to push investigations to their conclusions or to follow the exactness of method."[27]

[23] George B. Wood to Toner, July 4, 1866, *ibid.,* No. 94.
[24] See for examples, letters to Toner from Edward Alden of Randolph, Mass., July 28, 1866; Joseph Draper of Worcester, Mass., Sept. 23, 1867; J. M. Cooper of Lancaster, Pa., April 25, June 8, July 8, 1867; Ellsworth Eliot of New York, June 8, 1866; H. A. Ford of Leonardtown, Md., June 14, 1867; William M. Hiester of Reading, Pa., March 8, 1867; Robert S. Smith of Bound Brook, N. J., Oct. 9, 1866; W. C. van Bibber of Baltimore, Md., March 4, 1867; John L. Vandervoort of New York, Dec. 13, 1866; Claiborne Watkins of Little Rock, Ark., Oct. 9, 1869, Toner Papers, Nos. 8, 65, 74, 75, 76, 80, 91, 93.
[25] O. D. Palmer to Toner, Nov. 22, 1866, *ibid.,* No. 87.
[26] Toner to Joseph Carson, March 10, 1869, College of Physicians of Philadelphia.
[27] Toner, *Contributions,* 7.

Yet one wishes that his presentation had been less hasty and slipshod, better organized, more thoughtful, for he offered some generalizations most readers would like more light on. He noted, for example, that in colonial America the practice of the learned professions was apt to be combined in one person; he appreciated that sparseness of population was a reason for the lack of medical facilities; he included midwives in the medical profession, and named some; he explained at great length the distinction between physician and surgeon, and why in America both were called doctor; and he calculated the ratio of physicians to the general population, employing figures that have been widely accepted since.[28] Brief sections of the address were devoted to medical education, medical regulations, hospitals, physicians in the Revolutionary War, and similar topics; but the bulk of the monograph consisted of biographical notes on physicians, arranged by colony and state, often with only a fact or two about each: [29]

Dr. Cabin [Corbin] Griffin, born in Virginia of Welsh descent, practiced in Yorktown.
John Glover, having graduated at Harvard in 1650, went to Europe, where he received his medical degree at Aberdeen, Scotland. On his return he settled as a physician at Roxbury.
Thomas Oliver was in practice in Boston about 1640.

" You are certainly a wonderful digger in the mines of American medical lore," wrote Samuel D. Gross,[30] who read the little book at a sitting the same day it was delivered, " & deserve great credit for your painstaking labors. There are some very curious things in your brochure, which require to be closely studied to be fully appreciated." Then, turning to the subject of medical education, in which he was deeply concerned, Gross continued warmly:

If we could only raise the standard of education, preliminary & college, of our students, & make gentlemen of them all, how happy we both should be! The miserable wretches who now degrade our Schools, unwashed, with dirty nails, unkempt hair, slouched hats, with their hands in their pockets when they meet or pass a professor, are a disgrace to the profession, & injure the whole leven [?]. Surely there ought to be a remedy for all these *crimes*! Surely these *animals* ought to be kept out of a noble profession! If we could only have honest, competent boards of examiners, there might be some hope, but, as matters now are, there is no prospect of amelioration, no hope of improvement.

[28] *Ibid.*, 105-06.
[29] *Ibid.*, 12, 13.
[30] Gross to Toner, Jan. 2, 1875, Toner Papers, No. 78.

The *Annals of Medical Progress* was the first of three addresses or monographs which, between them, attempted to cover the whole history of medicine in the United States. The second, entitled *The Medical Men of the Revolution, with a Brief History of the Medical Department of the Continental Army,* was an address to the Alumni Association of Jefferson Medical College in March 1876. Announcing that his purpose was "not to eulogize—but to collect material and present a few facts from which history may be written," [31] Toner presented a full straightforward narrative of the medical department of the Continental Army, with some account of the Massachusetts provincial service that preceded it. The emphasis was on administrative history, with the facts drawn from the *Journals of the Continental Congress,* Peter Force's *American Archives,* the *Writings of George Washington,* the publications of John Morgan, and the records of provincial assemblies; but the monograph included many short biographical notes and sketches of several categories of physicians—the physicians- and surgeons-general, physicians who held civil office, and the like—and it ended with a list of 1200 names (which Toner said he forebore to read to his patient audience) of physicians and surgeons of the army and of medical men who served the American cause in other capacities. The list was not complete or accurate, but no one had ever compiled such a list before; and, refined and augmented, it remains useful to the present day.[32]

Hardly had Toner completed reading this address to the Jefferson alumni than he was called on for another—the concluding essay in his history of medicine in the United States.[33] The occasion was the International Medical Congress at the Centennial Exposition at Philadelphia in September. Toner's task, in this paper, was greater than any he had yet undertaken—to relate the progress of medicine in all 38 states of the Union, concentrating on the achievements and personalities of the century since 1776. It proved harder to learn about Missouri than Massachusetts medicine, and in some ways more difficult to determine the outstanding figures of the 19th than of the 18th century. To help in his preparation, Toner resorted again to a circular. He wrote scores, per-

---

[31] Toner, *Medical Men of the Revolution,* 6.

[32] *Ibid.,* 117-29. Compare Toner's list with that in Louis C. Duncan, *Medical Men in the American Revolution, 1775-1783* (Carlisle Barracks, Pa.: Medical Field Service School, 1931; reprinted New York: Augustus M. Kelley, 1970), 379-414.

[33] Toner, "Address on Medical Biography, delivered before the International Medical Congress at Philadelphia, September 5, 1876," *Transactions of the International Medical Congress* (Philadelphia, 1877), 91-137.

haps hundreds, of letters to his medical correspondents, asking them to name, preferably in order of distinction, the ten outstanding physicians and surgeons of their respective states.

The responses varied in interesting ways. The Boston physicians, for example, appear to have consulted together and agreed upon their list: Josiah Bartlett, Zabdiel Boylston, Edward Holyoke, James Jackson, James Lloyd, James Thacher, John Ware, John Warren, John C. Warren, and Benjamin Waterhouse.[34] (Toner dropped Zabdiel Boylston from the Massachusetts nominees because he fell outside the period; he added John Brooks, probably because of Brooks' distinguished record in military and public life.) But Ashbel Smith, sometime Texas minister to Great Britain and secretary of state of the Republic of Texas, declined for reasons of "delicacy" to make any selection. On the other hand, the Pennsylvanians were dismayed by the limitation to ten. "Remember Penn 'a has been always the seat of Medical Science in this country," warned William H. Egle, himself a historian as well as a physician, "and hence its bright galaxy of medical Stars." He sent Toner sixteen names, and added that there were as many more living and dead who were equally distinguished. "Now what shall I do with this array?" he demanded.[35] Alfred Stillé of Philadelphia, though protesting he had never taken any particular interest in medical history, sent along 13 names, which he was careful to arrange in alphabetical order.[36]

If Pennsylvania had too many outstanding physicians to choose from, other states had too few. Claiborne Watkins of Little Rock, for example, reminded Toner that Arkansas was not long removed from the wilderness. "I am convinced that there were many Physicians of real genius and eminence in their sphere, but alas! if I except isolated stories and

[34] See the replies of Nathan Allen of Lowell, Mass., April 10, 1876; Francis H. Brown of Boston, May 10, 1876; James R. Chadwick of Boston, May 2, 1876; Samuel A. Green of Boston, May 6, 1876; and Oliver W. Holmes of Boston, April 7, 1876, Toner Papers, Nos. 55, 70, 71, 78, 80. Holmes' letter is printed in an appendix to this paper.

[35] William H. Egle to Toner, April 22, 1876; Ashbel Smith to Toner, Aug. 26, 1876, Toner Papers, Nos. 75, 91.

[36] Alfred Stillé to Toner, April 4, 1876, ibid., No. 91.

Henry Bronson of New Haven, Conn., gave Toner the names of ten outstanding Connecticut physicians; but he was not happy about ranking them. "It is not possible to compare intelligently & successfully one talent, one attainment or accomplishment, one kind of skill or success, with another; great medl. scholarship & a limited practice with illiteracy combined with large experience & acknowledged skill, &c. I have no doubt the physicians of this State would be best satisfied with alphabetl. arrangement." To Toner, May 26, 1876, Toner Papers, No. 70.

traditions, their good deeds and accumulated experience died with them."
They had left no books, papers, lectures or other evidences of their study
and research to judge them by.[37] Illinois was also relatively young, too.
recently settled to have produced physicians of truly national reputation.
One who qualified was Daniel Brainerd. He was a man of undoubted
professional and scientific achievement, but it was regrettable, Nathan
S. Davis thought, that published biographical sketches said nothing about
his private character. " He was really one of the most purely selfish men
I ever knew, and during the last ten years of his life devoted more time
and thought to *real estate* speculation and money getting than to his profession. I do not mention this for you to repeat but simply to guard
against the commission of positive errors of statement." [38] Toner would
never have repeated Davis' characterization: the sketch of Brainerd appeared with no " positive errors of statement."

Dr. Daniel Brainerd, a native of New York, was a physician and surgeon of
distinction. He settled in Chicago as early as 1835, and soon acquired a leading
professional business, especially in Surgery. He was one of the founders of the
Rush Medical College, and long one of its professors. He contributed articles
of value to the Medical Journals, and to the Illinois State Medical Society's
Transactions. (b. 1812; d. Oct. 10, 1866.) [39]

The address opened with several pages of general medical history.
Dividing the century since 1776 into four quarters, Toner alluded briefly
to the influence of wars on medical and surgical knowledge in each period,
the impact of yellow fever and cholera epidemics, the benefits bestowed
by vaccination and anaesthesia, the founding of medical schools and the
proliferation of medical journals. He then described briefly the contributions of 20 outstanding physicians of the century just passed, and
offered 98 additional names without comment. The final portion of the
address, which was based on the replies to the letters Toner sent doctors
throughout the Union, contained the names of the outstanding physicians
of each of the 38 states. A comparison of the published text with the
nominations received shows that, with few exceptions, Toner included
in his lists every name that anyone proposed. In his original draft Toner
had written " formal biographies " of another hundred of " the most
eminent medical men of the United States." As it was, Toner's paper

[37] Claiborne Watkins to Toner, April 23, 1876, *ibid.*, No. 93.
[38] Nathan S. Davis to Toner, April 10, 1876, *ibid.*, No. 73.
[39] Toner, " Address on Medical Biography, " *loc. cit.*, 104-05.

ran to 47 closely printed pages; and the sketches were " necessarily "—
and, one feels mercifully,—" omitted for want of space." [40]

Two other biographical projects of Toner's should be mentioned. One
was the record of the Rocky Mountain Medical Association. This was
a social group, composed of 123 physicians, their wives, and a few non-
medical gentlemen who accompanied them from the east coast to San
Francisco in 1871 for the first meeting of the American Medical Association west of the Rocky Mountains. (Toner carried a letter of introduction to Brigham Young, but seems not to have used it.)[41] The members
held reunions during the annual Association meetings. In 1877 Toner,
as president, delivered an address with a title almost as long as the journey: " Some Observations on the Geological Age of the World, the
Appearance of Animal Life upon the Globe, the Antiquity of Man, and
the Archaeological Remains of Extinct Races found on the American
Continent, with Views of the Origin and Practice of Medicine
among uncivilized Races, more especially the North American Indians."
The address was based on wide, but superficial, reading; it revealed only
a library aquaintance with anthropology, archaeology, and paleontology.
Toner published it, together with the presidential addresses of former
years and a biographical dictionary of all the Rocky Mountaineers (prepared from data collected by a questionnaire) in a stout little volume
of 414 pages in 1877.[42] The second biographical project was to collect
data on each of the founders of the American Medical Association. Toner
consulted the widows, children, and colleagues of the deceased founders,
collected obituary notices from the medical and lay press, and, in the case
of survivors, succeeded in obtaining some informative personal recollections. Nathan S. Davis, for example, wrote a particularly interesting
account of his boyhood, education, early practice, and professional career
in Binghamton, N. Y., and Chicago.[43] And for 20 years Toner was
chairman of the Necrology Committee of the A. M. A., writing a good
many obituaries himself and compiling an alphabetical list of all ne-
crologies in the *Transactions* of the Association, which he printed as an
appendix to his own report of 1882.[44]

[40] *Ibid.*, No. 93.
[41] F. B. Steck to Young, May 7, 1871, Toner Papers, No. 8.
[42] Toner, *Address before the Rocky Mountain Medical Association, June 6, 1877*
(Washington, 1877).
[43] Nathan S. Davis to Toner, March 25, 1875, Toner Papers, No. 73.
[44] Fishbein, *History of the American Medical Association*, 623-24; Medical Society
of the District of Columbia, *Transactions*, n. s., 1897, *1*: 150, 155-56.

One reason why Toner could produce these prodigies of data—I have only hinted at his statistical studies, said nothing about his more modest historical addresses and compilations like that on theater fires, and will not mention the research and writing on George Washington which engrossed so much of the last 15 years of his life—was that he had a very large reference library of his own. From the time he came to Washington Toner was a tireless collector of medical books, concentrating on American imprints, medical journals, and the classics of the profession. He haunted the bookstores and junkshops, where his practice of buying old periodicals by the pound led some to think him undiscriminating, not realizing that he often found treasures in those bales of paper and used the rest for exchange. Even allowing for inflation, his purchases might excite the envy of a modern collector or librarian. A Providence, R. I., bookseller offered 50 volumes of the *Boston Medical and Surgical Journal* for 37-½ cents each. John Campbell of Philadelphia sold him Heberden's smallpox pamphlet, with Franklin's recommendation, for $10. From John K. Brady of Shakspear's Head in Baltimore, Toner bought Rush on the *Diseases of the Mind* for 75 cents, John Sappington's *Theory and Treatment of Fevers* for 20 cents, and inaugural dissertations and Philadelphia yellow fever pamphlets for 25 and 50 cents each. He lost William Smith's *Eulogium of Benjamin Franklin* at a Boston auction—his bid was $1.25, and it went for $1.75—but he acquired at the same sale a bundle of 26 medical pamphlets for $1.56. One dealer, after offering Toner four titles on the cholera epidemic of 1832, all from the library of John Redman Coxe, told him he had some early 18th-century books as well; these, he apologized, were " probably more curious than useful," but, he continued, as "negative evidence of the progress of the sciences," were " therefore of value." [45]

By 1870 Toner's library was growing at the rate of 800-1,000 volumes a year. A catalogue prepared in 1871 shows about 5,500 medical titles—Albinus, Bard, Elisha Bartlett, William Beaumont, Bichat, Boerhaave, Cullen, John Howard, William Hunter, Jenner, Morgagni, Samuel G. Morton, Rush, Lemuel Shattuck, Sydenham, Van Swieten, Vesalius.[46]

[45] Letters to Toner from Edward Barrington, April 23, 26, 1866; John K. Brady, Jan. 23, Feb. 6, 1866, Oct. 18, 1867; John Campbell, April 11, 1864; John P. Des Forges, July 10, 1866; O. F. Fassett, May 9, 1876; Frank J. O'Connor, March 12, 1878; Toner to C. F. Libby, Dec. 11, 1878, Toner Papers, Nos. 1, 6, 7, 76, 87.

[46] Dr. W. Lee, comp., A Catalogue of Medical Works in the Library of Dr. J. M. Toner, Arranged alphabetically by Authors (1871), Toner Papers, Box 159. In the same box are the supplements for 1872-78.

The collection also contained manuscript lecture notes taken by students of Benjamin Smith Barton, Boerhaave, Cullen, David Hosack, Valentine Mott, Alexander Monro, Benjamin Rush, and other teachers in both America and Europe;[47] and there were miscellaneous autograph letters: of physicians of the Revolution like James Craik, Silvester Gardiner, Edward Hand, Arthur Lee, James McHenry, Donald McLean, Johann David Schoepf, and James Thacher; and of public figures as well.

Laymen offered Toner books as gifts or to buy; executors asked about disposing of old books in the estates they administered. Such was his reputation that even professional librarians took his advice about how to store pamphlets properly and how to file loose sheets of paper.[48]

Toner's files were one of the wonderful features of the library. He had begun before 1860 to clip from the daily papers important state papers, public addresses, and reports of political events. He soon extended his coverage to necrology and biography. In the latter 1860s he engaged young women systematically to clip biographical sketches and notices of physicians from newspapers, medical journals, college alumni directories, and biographical dictionaries like Thacher's. Sometimes the clerks added bibliographical notes cut from library catalogues and booksellers' lists. From physicians, it was a short step to famous men of every age, nation, and profession. By 1880 a visitor to Toner's library might have been excused for believing his host had undertaken to compile a biographical register of a substantial portion of all the human beings who had ever lived.

Cut and trimmed with astonishing precision, the clippings were pasted on heavy paper sheets, about 8 by 10 inches in size; and these were filed alphabetically in several great wooden filing cabinets which Toner had constructed for the purpose. These cabinets of laboriously collected data survive in the Library of Congress to this day. One cabinet, containing 36 drawers, holds cards on which are mounted at least one fact about each of about 40,000 doctors. Two more cabinets of the same size—72 drawers in all—are filled with clippings on perhaps 80,000 non-physicians of every description: Chastellux, André Chénier, and Cheops are in close proximity. In addition Toner filled two large wooden foot-lockers to the brim with newspaper clippings on every imaginable topic;

[47] In Toner Papers, Nos. 142-46. Nos. 147-51 contain hundreds of printed dissertations, mostly of the 1830s and 1840s.
[48] Philosophical Society of Washington, *Bulletin,* 1885, *8*: 29; H. A. Ford to Toner, Aug. 24, 1888, Toner Papers, No. 76.

he sorted them roughly into small packets, but otherwise never got around to organizing them. Perhaps the most " finished " of the files of clippings are now to be found in some 40 small cases, designated by the Library of Congress " Toner Excerpts." These are longer newspaper stories, neatly mounted on heavy paper, the paper folded and stitched, with the title and source carefully written on the cover—the whole resembling a little pamphlet. If anything, the Excerpts are more varied than the other lots of clippings: in Case 25, for example, the first six items are an article headed " Air Fit to Breathe " from the Washington *National Republican,* 1884; the Proceedings of the International Medical Congress from the Washington *Star,* 1887; an article on " Street Car Rails : A New Method of Constructing Tramways," from the Washington *National Republican,* 1884; the Speech of Hon. Joseph Segar on the Disunion Issue, November 16, 1860, from the Washington *National Intelligencer,* 1860; an essay on Bedford, Pa., in the winter, from the Baltimore *Sun,* 1890; and a story on the origin of the Gridiron Club from the Washington *Evening Star,* 1889. Another clipping in this case of Excerpts is from a Washington paper of 1890, entitled " Seven of the Finest : Origin of the Police Force." [49]

Toner soon came to regard his library as a private obligation and a public service. During the cholera epidemic of 1865, for example, he circulated a list of the 68 books on the disease which he owned, offering to lend them to any doctor who might need them.[50] His fellow-physicians would stop by his house on Louisiana Avenue to borrow whatever they needed, leaving, if he was out, a note on their prescription form.[51] Soon Toner was receiving inquiries from out of town. William Pepper of Philadelphia, for example, required for a lecture on the reform of medical education the names of the medical schools actually in operation in the United States, with dates of founding. " I know of no one else in the country to whom I could apply with any chance of being directed where I can obtain this information," he explained. And when Pepper found he also wanted figures showing the number of physicians in Victoria, Australia, Toner got them, too.[52] He supplied one inquirer with a pack-

[49] Toner's three biographical file cabinets are in the Stack and Reader Division, Stack 29, Library of Congress. The " Excerpts " and the two chests of unsorted clippings are in the Rare Book Division, Library of Congress.

[50] *A Catalogue of Medical Works on Cholera, in the Library of J. M. Toner, M. D.* (Washington, 1865).

[51] A. F. A. King to Toner, April 27, 1874, Toner Papers, No. 83.

[52] William Pepper to Toner, July 22, Aug. 14, Oct. 21, 31, 1877, *ibid.,* No. 88.

age of pamphlets on the bad effects of graveyards, another with the names of all the practicing physicians in 15 southern and southwestern states, a third with the text of the missing title page of a history of the valley of Virginia. Even John Shaw Billings came to Toner for data that could not be found in the Surgeon General's Library.[53]

As the library grew Toner came to regard it not simply as a public service, but also as a national resource, which should not be dispersed at his death. Accordingly he offered it as a gift to any city that would erect a fireproof building to house it. Pittsburgh declined to accept it; Chicago failed to raise the money for the lot and building. Little Washington, Pa., which had a college with a new library building, expressed interest in receiving it.[54] So did the Library Company of Philadelphia, which had also just erected a huge building that could easily have absorbed the entire collection. Toner asked his friend Ainsworth R. Spofford, Librarian of Congress, about the Philadelphians' offer to take the collection. " The offer is a fair one, Doctor," Spofford replied, seizing his opportunity, " but the Library of Congress will do as well for you, I know." The prospect that " the pets of my life " would be safely deposited " under the Aegis of the Nation, for the future use and pleasure of those readers and students who shall come after us," appealed strongly to Toner;[55] and accordingly he gave his collection to the Library of Congress in 1882—the first such gift to the national library by a private citizen. Augmented by the books that came in after Toner's death, the collection numbered in 1897 nearly 25,000 volumes, as many pamphlets, and, it was estimated, nearly one million clippings.[56]

Because of his unquenchable passion for collecting, Toner's contemporaries called him " the Fact-Hunter."[57] He was indeed. He had seen enough incomplete, inaccurate, and misleading historical accounts to know that accurate data are indispensably necessary to sound historical writing of any kind. In a day when there were few biographical dictionaries,

[53] Inquiries from John Shaw Billings, April 12, 1876, Dec. 2, 1882; Josiah Drake, June 5, 1869; Edward Warren, Aug. 19, 1872; Stephen W. Wickes, Feb. 22, March 5, 1882, *ibid.*, Nos. 64, 74, 93, 94. When Toner could not supply S. Weir Mitchell with a copy of Sanctorius' *De erroribus in medicina evitandis,* the latter concluded the volume was not to be found in the United States. To Toner, Oct. 6 [1878], *ibid.,* No. 86.
[54] Joseph H. Little to Toner, Oct. 20, 1877; Nathan S. Davis to Toner, Dec. 25, 1878, *ibid.,* Nos. 73, 74.
[55]Toner to A. R. Spofford, March 19, 1882 (draft), *ibid.,* No. 1.
[56] *Report of the Librarian of Congress* (Washington, 1897), 37-38.
[57] Antisell, in Toner, *Address before the Rocky Mountain Medical Association,* 399-400.

bibliographies, or reliable biographies or histories; before Appleton, Kelly and Burrage, or the *Dictionary of American Biography* yet existed, Toner had to find out for himself who the doctors of two centuries had been. He addressed himself to his self-imposed task with unflagging industry; he urged others to follow his example; and his achievement was no mean one.

For his work Toner quickly realized he must have a library, as anyone must who wanted to do serious historical research and not merely repeat what others had published; and so a substantial part of his attention and substance were spent in building libraries and encouraging others to do so. His own collection, soon surpassing those of Samuel S. Purple of New York City and George J. Fisher of Sing Sing, N. Y.,[58] became one of the largest medical libraries in private possession. Long before he died in 1896 Toner assured its preservation by the nation. He was also a founder of the American Medical Association Library; he encouraged the Cambria County, Pa., Medical Society by bequeathing it his duplicates; and at the inauguration of the Columbia Historical Society he told his fellow-members firmly that in an institution like theirs a library was "a most urgent necessity."[59]

More than this, Toner had a sense of the importance of social history, which professional historians neglected in their concentration on political, constitutional, diplomatic, and military history. In his presidential address to the Columbia Historical Society in 1894 Toner stressed the importance of local and social history, the significance of every invention in the useful arts. In particular he urged his fellow-historians to identify the springs and water courses used by the first settlers, to locate the original shore lines and establish the elevations. These, of course, were aspects of public health that interested Toner professionally; but public health itself was an integral part of the broad view of history that he held.

In his appreciation of social history, his tireless compiling of data, his use of statistics, Toner could be considered a remote forerunner of the age of historiography that opened after his death. He thus displayed some of the excellent qualities of the amateur historian. Yet his work revealed some of the deficiencies of the amateur as well. Toner's methods were

[58] George J. Fisher to Toner, Nov. 11, 1882, Dec. 10, 1889, Toner Papers, No. 76.
[59] Toner, "Inaugural Address as President of Columbia Historical Society," (Washington) *Evening Star*, May 8, 1894, Toner Excerpts, Case 38, no. 10 (Rare Book Division, Library of Congress).

often careless, and he rarely asked the significance of the facts he gleaned so laboriously. All facts seemed to him of equal significance; he presented them with no discernible selection or organization and ,without interpretation. The rise of the medical profession in the United States after the middle of the eighteenth century, for example, illustrates a variety of intellectual movements and social processes; but Toner barely hinted at them, if, indeed, he was aware of them at all. The repeated disclaimers in his publications that they were only collections of data for others to use seem quite as much excuses for haste and incompleteness as expressions of scholarly modesty.

Like many amateurs, Toner attempted too much. Recognizing some important bibliographical needs and identifying gaps in knowledge of medical and public health history, he threw himself into the task of filling the deficiency with more energy and industry than intelligent direction. Toner might have compiled a reasonably complete biographical file on American doctors; but it was beyond his time and means to collect data on 100,000 others as well, from the Pharaohs to the present time. Ultimately the sheer labor of coping with the flood of clippings proved too much; he could no longer catalogue and index them. In 1882 Toner admitted to a correspondent that he had no thought of publishing the data he had collected.[60] Though in some respects a pioneer in medical history, Toner laid no foundations on which scholars coming afterwards could build; and his files and collections must have become as inaccessible to him as they are of little use to present-day scholars.

Though Toner's contemporaries might have recognized the basis of these criticisms, they would probably have judged them on the whole wrong-headed and ungracious. After all, Toner rescued a good many names from oblivion; he set out for the first time some of the basic facts of American medical history. His writings, addresses, and far-flung correspondence acquainted his fellow-physicians and others with the history of the profession and of an important part of the national history. His work was a starting point for the work of others. William A. M. Wainwright of Hartford, Conn., gratefully admitted that he had "cribbed" materials from Toner's "general History of the Profession" for an article of his own in 1887; while Paul F. Eve of Nashville, Tenn., told him that *Contributions to the Annals of Medical Progress* was " just what I needed in preparing my biographical sketches." [61] He encouraged many

---

[60] Toner to W. H. Bady, Aug. 20, 1882 (draft), Toner Papers, No. 64.

[61] Paul F. Eve to Toner, Dec. 17, 1874; W. A. M. Wainwright, Aug. 11, 1887, *ibid.*, Nos. 76, 93.

historians of medicine with gifts and loans of books, notes, and manuscripts. " I spent half the night devouring them," wrote John R. Quinan of Baltimore about the contents of one such parcel, "& felt as happy as a Boy with a few tickets to a Circus." [62]

For founding and encouraging libraries, for contributions as an officer of professional medical and public health associations, for published historical monographs, for making other medical historians as happy as schoolboys with tickets to a circus, Toner received generous and grateful recognition from his own generation. He may even be judged, by someone who will read his 75,000 letters preserved in the Library of Congress, to have deserved that reputation in the nineteenth century and our respect in the twentieth.

Appendix

Two Letters of O. W. Holmes to Joseph M. Toner, 1876

While preparing his address on American medical biography for the International Medical Congress at Philadelphia in 1876, Toner wrote Dr. Oliver Wendell Holmes, asking him to name the ten outstanding physicians in the history of Massachusetts. Upon receiving the reply (April 7), Toner sent Holmes copies of his own publications and asked for a copy of Holmes' lecture on medicine in Massachusetts. Holmes complied with the request (April 17) and added "a few words, somewhat confidentially," on the achievements of American medicine in the preceding century.

The letters are preserved in the Toner Papers, No. 80, in the Library of Congress. In the transcription of the letter of April 7, citations to biographical and other sources have been omitted.

Boston April 7th 1876

Dear Sir,

I have been consulting my memory and the medical biographies so as to enable me to make out a satisfactory list of ten names, as you requested, of Massachusetts physicians, deceased, proper to be mentioned as representatives of the profession, during the last century, among us. I think the list I give you is on the whole one which would be considered a fair one. I am of course prejudiced strongly in favor of my old instructors Dr. James Jackson and Dr. John Ware, yet I am

[62] John R. Quinan to Toner, March 25, 1881, *ibid.*, No. 88.

confident that both these names would be almost universally agreed upon as entitled to be classed with the elected ten representatives.

No.	Date of Birth	
1.	1680	Zabdiel Boylston. Introduced *inoculation* for small-pox into America.
2.	1728	Edward Augustus Holyoke. *The Centenarian.* Received a public dinner on his 100th birthday from the physicians of Salem & Boston. First President of the Massachusetts Med. Soc. An admired man and excellent physician.
3.	1728	James Lloyd. One of the best educated and most finished practitioners of his time. Thoroughbred, elegant, toryish, but the great Boston physician, surgeon etc. for nearly 60 years.
4.	1753	John Warren. Brother of Joseph Warren. Army surgeon. One of the earliest teachers of Anatomy. A founder, *the* founder, more than any other person of the Harvard Univ. Medical School.
5.	1754	James Thacher. Army surgeon in the Revolution. Author of Am. Med Biography—New Dispensatory—Observ. on Hydrophobia—Military Journal etc. etc.
6.	1758	Benjamin Waterhouse. Introduced *Vaccination* for small-pox into America. First Professor of Theory & Practice in Med. School of Harvard University.
7.	1777	James Jackson. Professor of Theory & Practice in Med. Sch. of H. U. from 1812 to 1836. The leading *medical* practitioner in Boston for many years. Author of Letters to a Young Physician etc.
8.	1778	John Collins Warren. Son of John Warren. Professor of Anatomy & Surgery etc. Med. Sch. of H. U. from 1815 to 1847. The leading *surgeon* in Boston for many years. Author of Surg. Obs. on Tumors and many other writings.
9.	1795	John Ware. Prof. of Th. & Pract. in Med. Sch. of H. U. from 1836 to 1858. Author of admirable papers on Delirium Tremens and Croup and of various other papers.
10.	1805	Elisha Bartlett (active in Lowell, Mass.). Professor in Coll. of Phys. & Surg. New York and in various other Institutions. Author of Philos. of Med. Science, A Treatise on Fevers. A remarkably candid, learned, philosophical and finished writer.

I have not mentioned Luther V. Bell, Samuel G. Howe, William G. Morton, Charles T. Jackson, Jeffries Wyman, all of whom had close relations with the medical profession, but were hardly known as medical practitioners.

If we could include the living I should name the venerable Dr. Jacob Bigelow Author of Am. Med. Botany, Sequel to the Dispensary, Nature in Disease and many other valuable books and papers; the originator of rural cemeteries (Mount Auburn) in this country, now nearly ninety years old, stone-blind, helpless in bed, but with a mind singularly bright and cheerful.

Henry J. Bigelow his son, whose treatise on Dislocations of the hip I am disposed to call the most original, thorough, and important contribution to surgical science (leaving out anaesthesis and perhaps ovariotomy) that I can now think of as having been made in this country.

As to etherization, they may fight about it as much as they like, it went forth to the world from the Massachusetts General Hospital and all the world knows the names connected with the first operation there which established it.

Dr Bowditch and Dr Morrill Wyman I believe share the credit of largely introducing paracentesis of the thorax in acute cases, but I know next to nothing about the matter, not having practised for more than twenty years.

It seems a pity that we cannot display the names of Dr Howe and of Jeffries Wyman on our State medical banner, but I suppose they would hardly be included.

Hoping that these hints may be a slight help to you, I am, my dear Sir

Yours very truly

O. W. HOLMES

P. S. I suppose of course you can get at the Transactions of the Mass. Med. Society. Also that you have or can get at my Lecture before the Mass. *Historical* Society on the history of Medicine in Massachusetts. I take it for granted that you have everything in your great Library at Washington and that Dr Billings knows all that has been written since Chiron took a pen in his hoof.

2d Postscript. I have not included *Nathan Smith,* because though he was born & educated in Massachusetts, he taught & practised mostly in other states.

Boston April 17th 1876

My dear Sir,

I think after seeing the publications of your own which you have kindly sent me, and for which I return my thanks, I may say that you have no occasion to ask any hints from me. I send you the Lecture I referred to, from which you may possibly glean something, and which at least will show you my way of treating a subject in some degree like that which you have to deal with.

I am going now to say a few words, somewhat confidentially, as it appears to me that you are one of the few Americans who like facts better than rhetoric.

A great many good, honest, sensible doctors, of fair intelligence and some professional knowledge, who have worked faithfully and devotedly in their calling and deserve to be held in honorable remembrance, we have doubtless had in this country. But our original contributions to medical science have been of very moderate amount, unless we include *dentistry*, where I suppose our countrymen have done a good deal. Take Anatomy, for instance. How utterly insignificant do our contributions seem! We live chiefly on the reputation of ' Horner 's muscle ' so called, though Duverny seems to have described it in 1749. * In physiology we have done a little better since the recent days of physiological laboratories. There

---

* I ought not to forget Morton's ' Crania Americana.' His ' Anatomy ' is not what we might have expected of him.

may have been important contributions to practical medicine, but if I were asked point blank to name the six chief ones among them—apart from those respectable and useful compilations of which our country has been prolific, I should blush and stammer and write post haste to you or Dr Billings to know what they were.

No doubt we have done much better in Surgery. The magnificent army reports are perhaps its best monuments. Perhaps I might go further and say that *medical* as well as surgical *statistics* were the best things we had to show with the exception of very few really novel and ingenious practical innovations.

Anaesthetics constitute our chief claim in the eyes of the civilized world. I wish, if you refer to that, you would expose the contemptible way in which Simpson attempted to rake into his own crib the whole credit of their introduction, in the 8th edition of the Encyc. Britannica. Look out the different heads ' Anaesthetics, ' ' Ether, ' etc. & then look at Chloroform. (I am writing my recollection for the references.)

I have no doubt that with surgery and medical and surgical Statistics a fair show enough can be made. But I should not want to claim too much, or stretch the necks of native geese, otherwise quite respectable, to make them out swans, as in my opinion Gross had done in his recent review, notwithstanding that I myself came in for a share of his cartload of flattering epithets. Of all things I would avoid spread-eagle-ism in medicine. Its useful ministrations, not its show, not the ' brilliancy ' of jabbering professors, are what it has to contemplate with satisfaction. I have made too many fine phrases myself to throw stones at other rhetoricians, but for all that I have the most intense digust for the provincial exaggerations with which our countrymen are infested as with a disease—*morbus pedicularus*—acari—ascarides—or what you will—something which keeps up an itching only to be allayed by the application of superlatives.—On talking over these matters with Dr. Edmund H. Clarke (who has long been confined to his house with an internal ulcerative rectum—which does not seem to get better) he spoke of our *army hospital improvements,* which were so much thought of by the Germans in their late war. He also referred to Drs. Bowditch & Wyman's operation of *paracentesis thoracis,* to which I think I called your attention in my other letter. He also called to my notice the way in which Dr Gross had slighted Dr Bigelow's Treatise on Dislocations of the Hip—a first class contribution to surgery as the European surgeons have found out.

Believe me dear sir, Yours very truly

O. W. HOLMES

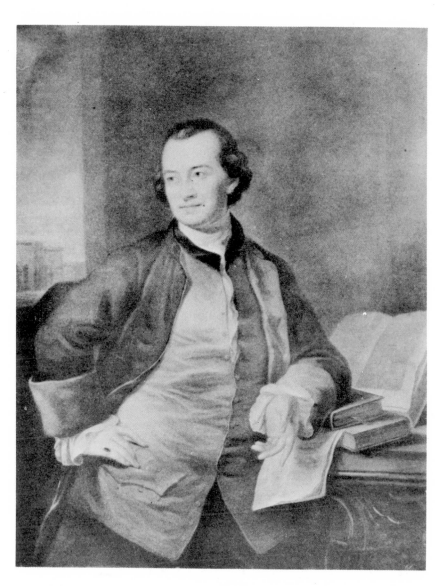

JOHN MORGAN

JOHN MORGAN, FOUNDER OF THE
MEDICAL SCHOOL

Adventures on the Trail of his Biography

WHEN it was first suggested that I write a biography of John Morgan I had no clear idea where the task would lead. I knew, of course, that Morgan was the founder (at the University of Pennsylvania) of the first medical school in America and that he was director of medical services in Washington's army. I had read his *Discourse upon the Institution of Medical Schools in America*, which is a milestone in the history of medical education; and I knew that the journal of his Grand Tour had been carefully edited and privately printed in a small edition. A few of his letters, preserved in libraries in Philadelphia, I had read for another purpose some time before. But almost all that I really knew about John Morgan was that no one had ever written his biography; and I believed he deserved to have one done.

For John Morgan appears in all the histories of American medicine, science, and culture, frequently, to be sure, not as a distinct personality, but always as a symbol of the maturing culture of colonial America. A member of the first graduating class of the University, then the College of Philadelphia (1757), after service as a surgeon with provincial troops in the French and Indian War, he went abroad to study medicine. In London he lived with John Hunter and was a student of anatomy under Dr. William Hunter; at Edinburgh, where he received his M.D. degree in 1763, his teachers thought him the very model of a medical student, with sound assurance of a great career. He travelled through Holland with James Boswell, famous biographer of Dr. Samuel Johnson; he visited Italy with the Duke of York; and he spent a lively evening with Voltaire at Ferney. When he returned home in 1765 he had such a reputation that Philadelphians are said to have rushed to the windows when he passed, just so they could say they had seen him.

Within a fortnight he was elected professor of the theory and practice of medicine in the College, and a month later delivered the memorable *Discourse*, which called for standards of medical education and practice so high that they were not practicable in American society for more than a century. For fourteen months in 1775-1777 he headed the medical services of the Revolutionary Army before Boston and New York. The conditions of the military hospitals were bad, though this was not his fault alone, and the Congress summarily removed him from office. He spent two years securing a vindication and two more pressing charges against his successor. As a veteran of the Indian war, he was interested in bounty lands; as a member of the American Philosophical Society, in balloons and the bones of prehistoric monsters. He encouraged domestic manufactures as varied as silk and iron; and among the letters of introduction which the artist Copley carried to Italy in 1773 were half a dozen from Morgan. Such a man, it seemed to me, deserved a biography.

Startled, perhaps, by the warm encouragement of the publisher, I begged a few weeks to make a brief survey of materials. Very little, I quickly found, had been written about Morgan; and most of this was a repetition of something said before. Benjamin Rush's *Eulogy*, delivered in 1789, and James T. Flexner's lively chapter in *Doctors on Horseback*, published in 1937, stood at two extremes in time. Between there were Dr. George W. Norris' *Early History of Medicine in Philadelphia* and Joseph Carson's *History of the Medical Department of the University of Pennsylvania*, but very little else of first value. There were two pamphlets of Morgan's authorship, some broadsides, several communications to the American Philosophical Society, and a number of letters in the Philadelphia press. A few weeks sufficed to find most of this material. It was not much. It was clear that if a full account of Morgan's life was to be written at all, I must find my way to Morgan's letters and papers —if, indeed, such manuscripts actually existed.

I was almost certain there was no single great collection of Morgan manuscripts in any library, as there is of Washington's at the Library of Congress and of Rush's at the Library Company of Philadelphia. This is partly because most of Morgan's library was destroyed during the American Revolution; partly because at the end of his life, when he was sick and discouraged, he destroyed many papers himself. Morgan letters were likely to be widely scattered and no library would own more than a few.

With the Philadelphia libraries I was already pretty well acquainted. The Historical Society of Pennsylvania has Morgan's earliest letter, a description of Philadelphia filling with troops for the frontier campaign of 1756 and Major Washington having business with the Assembly; and the last account of Morgan, Benjamin Rush's first-hand description of his lonely death, is at the Library Company. In the Medical School he founded is the original of Morgan's Italian journal, while the official records of the Trustees respecting the Medical Department are in the custody of the Secretary of the University. I had to learn what other libraries held. Inquiries to the historical societies of Massachusetts, New York, Maryland, and Virginia, for example, brought replies which were hardly encouraging. Most reported no Morgan letters at all; the others had but one or two; and two of these proved to be only notes about the rental of a stable on Cypress Street, Philadelphia.

Perhaps I ought to have stopped here. But it was at precisely this point that the work began to take on the fascination which marks so many research problems. Surely there is nothing unique in this story of John Morgan's biography—every incident in it can be repeated by a thousand other biographers. Nor was the dull grubbing of scholarship transmuted here by invisible inks or croquet boxes into some timeless task. But I liked it all the same, and my heart beat faster every time I learned something new about Morgan. The search was the more intriguing, I think, just because there were so few letters and each one I found represented a kind of minor triumph. In time I located manuscripts in places as far from home as Honolulu and Amsterdam. I found them in places as obvious as the Library of Congress and as unexpected as the offices of an old English drug firm. Occasionally letter-writing and leg-work were rewarded by a rich cache of letters, as at Prestonfield in Scotland; but more often there was disappointment: only the other day, for example, a Morgan descendant reported that in his collection of family papers, the envelope marked John Morgan is empty.

Frequently, as in this case, descendants could offer me little help; yet some of my pleasantest associations have been with them. Actually, they are not descendants of John Morgan, who had no children, but of his brother George. Early in my work I learned who they are from the bibliography in a life of George Morgan by Dr. Max Savelle. One of these descendants, the late Robert R. Reed of Washington, Pa., was seriously ill when I wrote asking for an appointment. His wife replied that I had better send her my questions in writing. A few days later she sent me her husband's answers, including the names and addresses of most of the members of the family who owned Morgan papers.

By Mr. Reed I was directed to another Morgan descendant. I shall not forget the evening I spent with him at his club in Boston. Before the last war he inherited a bundle of family papers, but, busy with his own work, he had never inspected them. After a comfortable dinner we withdrew to a small table to open the package. There were over a hundred letters and documents, principally George Morgan's, as I suspected they would be, but several were John's. Among these I found a list of all the household furnishings he sold in 1788, and one-half of the inventory of his personal property in 1789—documents of no cosmic significance, to be sure, but important when they are all you have! My excitement was unsuppressed as we unfolded each old paper, but I believe my host enjoyed that evening even more than I. It was past two when I returned to my hotel.

To locate Morgan letters in private hands was the most difficult task. There is simply no way of knowing what letters may be in an autograph collection only twenty miles away. Once I examined for Morgan items the hundreds of autograph sales catalogues preserved at the Historical Society of Pennsylvania. Catalogue descriptions are better than nothing; sometimes letters are quoted in whole or in part; while in a few catalogues someone had noted the names of the purchasers of every letter. Several of these pencilled notes read "Pepper." This, I knew, should be Dean William Pepper of the University's Medical School.

Dean Pepper was all kindly interest when I met him one afternoon in the library of the Medical School. He was amused to learn how I knew what he had bought at autograph sales 40 years before. Most of his Morgan letters, he explained, had already been presented to the University; but he pointed to one which hung on the wall of the Dean's Office and directed that it be transcribed for me; and he showed me a valuable set of student notes taken in Morgan's time at the Pennsylvania Hospital. When I left him he warned me not to dawdle, for he wanted to read the book. "I am an old man," he added, "and can't wait long." Two weeks later he was dead.

Knowing my Morgan interest, friends have often directed me to manuscripts in private hands. In this way I met the late Dr. Robert P. Elmer, a remarkable man, at whose home I spent two full days reading the notes of medical lectures taken in Philadelphia by his ancestor Jonathan Elmer, who was one of Morgan's first students. In a lively letter he welcomed me to his home, provided I promised not to despoil these ancient volumes of their title-pages as another visitor had done. I replied in the same vein, that he might search me for knives and razors as I crossed his threshold. Anything as crude as these tools, he retorted scornfully, he never imagined; he referred to the criminal use of moistened string or thread. (You soak a string well between teeth and cheek, then place it close to the binding margin on the page you want to remove. Now close the volume for a minute, thus moistening the page along the line of the string. Take the page firmly between thumb and forefinger and pull it gently from the book. The page should come out easily, and can be swiftly concealed beneath your working notes.) * At other times Morgan letters have come unsolicited, as when, at the close of a meeting where I spoke on Morgan, a gentleman approached and promised to send me a transcript of a Morgan letter he owned as soon as he returned home to Honolulu. Five months later it arrived, interesting instructions to Aaron Burr about Morgan's land-holdings in western New York. Other letters of this correspondence with Burr are at the Library of Congress and Yale University.

Few men made a greater effort in my behalf than a French scholar I never met. I was given his name as that of a historian who might know where to find the records of the old Royal Academy of Surgery of Paris, of which Morgan was a corresponding member. Almost by return mail I had his own careful transcripts of the relevant portions of the minutes of the Academy, and a few days later he sent me microfilms of other records. He expressed regret for the delay and for any illegibilities, explaining that, as the transcripts were made in a period when the French Communists were on strike and there was no electricity, he had copied the minute books by candlelight.

Slowly as my files filled with notes the picture of the man Morgan began to take shape. For a moment I had the wildly romantic thought that he had had an attachment to Angelica Kaufmann, whom he knew at Rome; but my imagination soon cooled before the hard fact that the self-portrait which Angelica painted for him hung for years under the gaze of Mrs. Morgan in their Philadelphia home. Mrs. Morgan's letters to her husband, written when they were separated by the war, are warm and loving; there is even a poem singing the joy which she experiences

> . . . in possessing
> The greatest of all earthly Blessing,
> United to the Man I Love
> whose every Word, and action prove
> him the most worthy of his sex . . .

On the whole, however, though many of his early friends seem to have held him in warm affection, Morgan emerged as a formal, proud, and even jealous man, more respected by his fellows than loved. Only two or three anecdotes survive in which he appears, and then not always to his credit; while his letters are all so correct

---

* This works beautifully on pages of the *Saturday Evening Post*. I cannot speak for eighteenth century paper.

that I cannot raise so much as a smile by the cheap but effective device of quoting bad spelling and awkward grammar.

Several problems still vex me. One, as I have intimated, is Morgan's character; and this is probably the key to several others. I know surprisingly little about his medical work. To a physician interested in medical history I once spoke enthusiastically of Morgan the connoisseur of art, Morgan the patron of learning, Morgan the balloonist, Morgan the soldier. "Don't forget, young man," he reminded me, "that after all John Morgan was a physician." I remember this advice, but I have found relatively little evidence of the fact. Apparently only one record book of his practice survives, and this covers the last years of his life when he was admittedly not busy. I am troubled by the problem of who founded the Medical School and why Morgan seemed to ignore Dr. William Shippen, with whom he had jointly planned for the Medical School when they were in Edinburgh. As late as the fall of 1764 they were apparently still on good terms; yet by this time Morgan had completed the draft of the *Discourse* in which he speaks of Shippen as though the two were strangers. And, finally, I am still hewing my way, and often getting lost, in that four-year-long controversy between Morgan and Shippen over the conduct of the medical department in the Revolution, trying to fix the rights and wrongs and establish a few facts amid a wilderness of charges and counter-charges.

Sometimes a relatively small fact proved to have seemingly endless ramifications. Morgan's collection of mastodon's bones began as a footnote to the biography; it ended as a little chapter in international scientific relations in the eighteenth century. It all began with an entry in the diary of John Adams, declaring that one night in 1774, at the home of Dr. John Morgan for dinner, he was shown by his host "some bones of an animal of enormous size found on the banks of the river Ohio." There was no reason to believe these bones had a special story; I learned nothing more about them; and I tentatively concluded with respect to them that they were merely more evidence of Morgan's interest in natural history. But from Charles Coleman Sellers' life of Charles Willson Peale I learned that Peale had made some drawings of the bones of a mastodon for a German doctor in 1784. A footnote sent me to a publication of the New York State Museum; and I looked up the original Peale diary on which Mr. Sellers' biography rested. The bones which Peale drew did indeed belong to Morgan; and the German doctor's name was Michaelis. The *Index-Catalogue of the Surgeon General's Library* produced a reference to an article on Michaelis and nerve-regeneration; this referred in turn to Michaelis' letters from America which were printed in the German *Chirurgische Bibliothek* between

1779 and 1784. In one of these letters the German told how he visited Morgan to inspect the collection of old bones, how he found them in a corner, some of the dirt in which they originally lay still clinging to them, and how he had cleaned them before he could examine them. My tentative conclusion about Morgan's lively interest needed revision.

Meanwhile one of the Carnegie *Guides* to materials on American history in European libraries indicated several Morgan letters at the University of Amsterdam. I ordered photostats. Addressed to the eminent Dutch anatomist Petrus Camper, the letters related to the sale of Morgan's collection to Camper. Searching now for data on Camper, I found an invitation to attend the celebration of the 150th anniversary of his death in the spring of 1939 at the University of Groningen. As part of the celebration a Camper exhibition would be held. I wrote to Groningen for a catalogue of this exhibition, if any had survived the war. The catalogue listed drafts of several letters from Camper to Morgan. The correspondence on the subject of the sale of the collection was now complete. Camper, it appeared, studied Michaelis' pictures and reproduced them in an article published in the transactions of the Imperial Academy of Science of St. Petersburg. Subsequently Baron Cuvier studied the Peale pictures, then asked Camper's son to re-examine the Morgan bones; and on the basis of young Camper's report Cuvier was able to state categorically in 1806 that the mastodon was a distinct and separate species. To make the story complete, I should add that an inquiry to the professor of natural history at Groningen produced photographs of the bones which Dr. Morgan showed John Adams that night so long ago, now carefully preserved in The Netherlands.

I took John Morgan to Great Britain with me in the summer of 1949. Though I had other tasks, I never failed to search for Morgan in the manuscript catalogues of the libraries there; and there were days when Morgan occupied my whole time. Except at Prestonfield I found nothing of great importance, but each unrelated fact I turned up in this gleaning will add precision to a portrait which still has its hazy spots. Such a fact was the contemporary copy of Morgan's post-mortem findings in a case of hydrophobia at the Royal Infirmary of Edinburgh, which I found in the Medical Society of London. And, of course, a few places, where I might have found more data, were destroyed—St. Thomas' Hospital, for example, where so many eighteenth century American students of medicine walked the wards, had been cruelly damaged in the blitz.

Everywhere in Britain, whether or not there was something to show me, I met with a friendly reception. The library of the Royal College of Physicians of London, for example, was not yet restored to order after its wartime evacuation from Pall Mall. It was not normally open to the public, I was told politely; but, as I was a visitor from a great distance who could not conveniently return next month or next year, I was shown the catalogue and assured that every effort would be made to find me anything I might want. This cordial consideration I found everywhere; perhaps it was this that made the task of using series upon series of printed, bound catalogues (instead of trays of cards) less appalling than I feared.

One British librarian I recollect with special pleasure because he enjoyed some quiet amusement at the expense of the Americans and so provided me with a good story. I had gone to the library of the War Office to learn something about the organization of British army medical services at the time Morgan was in the provincial forces. Looking at me curiously, one of the staff drew down a book which he said was the best thing on the subject, done, he added, "by one of your own men." It was E. E. Curtis' *Organization of the British Army in the American Revolution*, a Yale Press publication. I had read it as an undergraduate and it had only three pages on the hospital. At the end of the day, however, I was directed to a volume of War Office Papers in the Public Record Office.

Next morning I was in Chancery Lane. It was my first experience with the Public Record Office. As I entered the building I may have thought I should find some data there; I am sure I never expected to go away with an amusing anecdote. At once I was asked if I had a reader's ticket. I had not, but thinking I would be directed to an office just down the hall, asked where I must go for one. I must return to the American Embassy, I was told; and ask the Embassy to write a letter to the British Foreign Office, requesting the Foreign Office to write a letter to the Master of the Rolls, requesting that official to grant me permission to use the Record Office. I understood that this is the way things are sometimes done in England, made no protest, but asked only how long this process usually required. "About two weeks," came the casual reply. "But," the librarian added cheerfully, noting the look of dismay for which I am now almost certain he was waiting, "for Americans we have a faster way." "What is that?" I inquired hopefully. "We telephone," was the answer.

And telephone they did. I returned to the Embassy, where an efficient young woman, after listening to a story she had heard from many others, phoned the Foreign Office. The officer at the other end must have protested. "But this *is* important," I heard her explain patiently; "we never ask you to telephone unless it is important." By the time I returned to the Record Office an hour later it was all arranged. But the letters followed the phone conversations;

and ten days after I had completed my search in the War Office Papers, I received a neat, formal note from the Master of the Rolls granting me permission to use the Public Record Office.

Morgan spent two years at Edinburgh, where he received the freedom of the city and was often a guest in the homes of some of the best known citizens. I believed there must be some material there. At the very least I hoped to learn where he lived—a photograph of the old building, if it stood, might make an interesting illustration for the book. I knew simply that he roomed with a Mrs. Stewart near the Netherbow Port. The *Edinburgh Directory* of the period was of no help—it showed half a dozen persons named Stewart who were, in the Scots' phrase, "room-setters," and more than one lived in the vicinity of the ancient eastern gateway. I gave up the search, and was content with a print of the Netherbow Port itself. But a few months later the cataloguers in the Historical Society of Pennsylvania turned up two new Morgan letters which answered my questions: one to Morgan in care of Mrs. Stewart in World's End Close; the other from Mrs. Stewart herself.

The door of the Royal College of Physicians in Queen Street was always locked and the bell resounded hollowly in the cavernous distance. But the librarian was a lively man with an engaging grin, who had made American history his special hobby. He delighted to produce the minutes of the College and other papers which recorded Morgan's election as a licentiate and Fellow. I fear I showed him no mercy as I sent him off for one volume after another. He produced them all, and some more besides; and I spent several dusty days poring over the 25 or more volumes of the correspondence of Morgan's Edinburgh teacher William Cullen. But these letters were almost all of a strictly professional character; I found only one from Morgan, but several from Morgan's fellow-Americans presented a warm report of the great Scottish teacher by his admiring students.

The afternoon at Prestonfield was the climactic moment of my search for Morgan materials in Scotland. I marvel now that I did not miss it entirely. Certainly I had not been very bright about it; I was almost reluctant to follow my nose where it pointed. I knew that John Morgan was well acquainted with Sir Alexander Dick, president of the Royal College of Physicians of Edinburgh, a country gentleman whose estate was Prestonfield near Edinburgh, a man of such parts that his friend Boswell actually began to prepare his biography before he finally settled on Dr. Johnson. I always inquired for Dick papers, thinking that among them some Morgan letters might be found. My first inquiry in an Edinburgh library elicited a reference to the *Dictionary of National Biography* and a promise to think on my problem. Others told me flatly there were no Dick papers; and at least two persons who ought to have known informed me that Prestonfield was at present occupied by tenants, that the owner lived on the Continent. I confess I made no effort to visit Prestonfield; I was busy with other things and kept telling myself that even if papers were hidden away in the attic the tenants would not know of them or, if they did, could not let me see them.

I was planning to leave Edinburgh on a Monday to spend a few days with friends in England before sailing home. On the preceding Saturday I was visiting several librarians who had been especially helpful, to say good-bye. The gentleman who had promised a month before to think on my problem now asked me if I knew *Curiosities of a Scots Charta Chest*, which contained material on Alexander Dick. I had never heard of the book, and added that I was not so much interested in Dick as in his American friends; but, as he was insistent, I walked across to the National Library and called for the volume. My eyes caught Morgan's name in the index. The book contained casual quotations from five or six letters from Morgan to Dick. I fairly shouted.

Where, I demanded of my librarian friend, are the originals of these letters. They existed 50 years before; they must surely be somewhere now. He thought that the Dick family solicitors might help and turned to a directory of the solicitors and land agents of the noble and country families of Britain. The solicitors of that member of the Dick family, who lived in France, were an Edinburgh firm. It was now almost 12 o'clock noon, but I hastened into Melville Street nonetheless, knowing that many things are tolerantly forgiven the energetic Americans. I spoke to one of the partners. The firm did handle the Dick estate, but he suggested that I return Monday to see his partner whose special responsibility it was. I thought it worthwhile to delay my departure for England, so I sent off some telegrams and presented myself in Melville Street again on Monday afternoon.

There I was taken in charge by the firm's cashier, an elderly man who reminded one of a Dickens' character, who explained that the gentleman I wanted to see had been detained. Would I return next morning at ten? Frankly I felt there was little prospect of finding anything and, moreover, I wanted to see my friends in England. We were by this time in one of the offices. I asked the cashier if he knew that there were in fact such papers as I inquired for. He was such a model of Scots' probity that he would only answer that I ought to return next day. As I turned to leave the room I saw piled against the wall, almost from floor to ceiling, dozens of great metal document chests. On eight or nine the name "Dick" was painted! I assured him I would return next day, and sent off more telegrams.

The solicitor, when I called next morning, was interested and sympathetic, but he thought I would find nothing except legal papers in his possession. I agreed this was probably true and we looked into several of the boxes for confirmation. But, as I turned to go, he asked, half-puzzled, why I had not gone out to Prestonfield. I gave him my reason, that there was no one there who could help. "But," he countered, "Mrs. Dick-Cunyngham lives there." It was my turn to be astonished. This was someone I had never heard of. That afternoon I was at Prestonfield.

As I walked up the tree-lined drive leading to the fine old seventeenth-century house where Sir Alexander entertained Morgan and Rush and Benjamin Franklin, with Arthur's Seat towering grandly just behind, I wondered whether I ought not to have left Edinburgh the day before as I planned. Surely nothing would come of this, and I should be lucky to spend as much as a night near Manchester with a friend of war days in Italy. There was no movement about the house as I approached, but the door was open and, as there was no bell, I was well into the hall before I attracted any attention. Yes, Mrs. Dick-Cunyngham replied to my questions, there were some old papers; she knew nothing of them herself; but if I could wait until her daughter returned from town, she might be able to help. We visited pleasantly for nearly an hour, walking through the house and grounds, chatting about Dick, market-gardening, and the Labor government. When the daughter returned, I recited my list of inquiries again; of all the names I mentioned—Franklin, Rush, Morgan, for examples—only Morgan's was familiar. She disappeared but returned in a moment with a great wooden bowl filled with eighteenth century letters. "I think there are some Morgan letters here," she said, dumping the contents into my lap.

There were indeed! Neatly tied up in a blue envelope marked "Dr. Morgan of Philadelphia" were nine letters. Except for those brief quotations in the *Scots Charta Chest* none had been read outside the family. And what wonderful letters they were, some of the best Morgan ever wrote—three from Paris, one from Rome, three from Philadelphia. They told many things I had not known, about his studies in Paris, about the Grand Tour, about his medical classes at Philadelphia, about the American Philosophical Society. I cannot say that any single group of Morgan letters is the most important; but I almost believe the Prestonfield letters are.

Mrs. Dick-Cunyngham, all friendly efficiency, offered me her desk so that I might go to work at once. Her daughter made the suggestion I wanted to make; she stuffed the letters into her purse and next morning we had them all photostated in town. I received the prints in London the night before I sailed.

NOTES & DOCUMENTS

ADAM CUNNINGHAM'S ATLANTIC CROSSING, 1728

THE hardships and hazards of ocean travel in the 18th century were accepted with such equanimity that accounts of even the most dangerous passages were often expressed with a detachment that makes them all the more moving. Such a record is Adam Cunningham's, made during a voyage from Scotland to Virginia in 1728 in a vessel carrying indentured servants to America.

Cunningham's journal of that voyage is a catalogue of terrors and sufferings. The captain was a drunkard who knew so little of his business that the crew once locked him in his cabin during a storm and managed the vessel themselves. The indentured servants broke open the wine chest one night and drank off three dozen bottles. The bread was consumed, the water turned foul and then gave out, until the crew were too weak from hunger and scurvy to do their duty, and the captain had to beg each passing vessel, often vainly, for a few provisions. One of the men fell overboard; for some days thereafter sharks followed the ship hungrily as it wandered along the aimless course the captain "charted." A tropical hurricane carried off the masts while all the servants and half the crew cowered helplessly below decks. Approaching its destination, the ship sailed past the Chesapeake Capes, and adverse winds delayed its return. When it got within the Capes at last, by either the captain's ignorance or his bravado, the ship ran aground, and the emaciated survivors of six harrowing months at sea stumbled ashore at last.

Little is known of Adam Cunningham, either in Scotland or in America. He was the son of Sir William Cunningham of Capring-ton in Scotland and a brother of Alexander Cunningham, who succeeded to the baronetcy of Prestonfield as Sir Alexander Dick.[1]

---

[1] On the Cunningham family generally see Hon. Mrs. Atholl Forbes, *Curiosities of a Scots Charta Chest, 1600-1800* (Edinburgh, 1897).

Adam studied medicine, probably in Edinburgh, perhaps also at Leyden, as his brother did; but he took no degree. The young men's father, old Sir William, once contrasted Alexander's " filial and kindly concern" with Adam's very different behavior; and there is reason to believe that Adam was at best heedless and unkind, and at worst that he went to the colonies because he got into some scrape at home.[2] He sailed from Scotland on April 4, 1728, with the intention of settling in Virginia as a physician.

May 5. Fair clear weather. We steer to the NW and make pretty good way, running twixt 6 and 7 knots per hour.[3]

May 6. The wind due west, so we steered NNW or NW and by N. About 4 in the afternoon we spied a sail and the master taking his glass, could make nothing of her. About one hour [afterwards] she came within one hundred and fifty yards [of us, fired a] sharp shot, which brushed by our broad side, [afterwards] flying out a white ensign. We now thought [she took us for] a French pirate or an Algerine man. Therefore [we presently] struck and hauled in our colors; but when we spoke them, we found [they] were French men and their Captain drunk, who out of bravado had fired at us, seeing we were defenceless. [From the] same to

May 18 we had generally calms. About the [22] we saw a ship on our larboard side about 4 miles distance from us. It being then break of day and our Captain much in liquor, we did not much care for speaking to them, but our Captain would speak to them and it being then a very rolling sea, as we were coming very nigh to speak them, a heavy wave dashed our ship against her bowsprit, which broke part of it, and we would not have escaped damage, had it not been by the dexterity of our steersman. The ship was a Frenchman lately come from Newfoundland load with codfish. We were then about the latitude of 47-00.

May 23. The winds still proving contrary, we resolved to steer to the S, and continued doing so until June 2, when the wind shifted to SW; then were were obliged to steer NW and WNW, which we continued for 6 days. About this time the servants aboard that were to be transported, broke open our wine chest and stole about 3 dozen of our wines, which was a great loss to us, our water beginning to smell. They were lashed to the pump and whipped with a cat-of-nine tails. [June] 8 the wind shifts to NE and we steer [W and] continue so to the 14. We now

---

[2] Sir William Cunningham to Alexander Cunningham, Edinburgh, December 19, 1724. This letter, those cited below, and Adam Cunningham's journal are in the possession of Mrs. Dick-Cunnyngham and her daughter Mrs. Janet Oliver of Prestonfield, Edinburgh, by whose kind permission they are presented here.

Spelling, capitalization, and punctuation have been modernized.

[3] The first two pages of the journal, containing the record of the first month at sea, are lost.

plainly see the [Captain's] humor, for he gets himself drunk every night, never minding the course of the ship; and seeing our liquors beginning to run scarce, the supercargo and I take our own shares, leaving the other to him to do as he pleased, which he had not above 8 days before it was finished.

June 14. The wind at W and continues from W by N to W by S most part of this month. Here we had more wine stole from us, for which the principal rogue was hanged up at the main yard's arm and then plunged into the sea for 3 or 4 times successively; the rest were whipped at the main yard [mast?]. We are now almost out of liquor and therefore very sparing, our water being very loathesome to drink.

July 1. Exceeding hot weather, we being now in the latitude of 36-45. The weather very calm. Our men are so fatigued with heat they can scarce handle the sails, and our water very bad.

July 3. Spied a brig about 2 leagues ahead. We immediately hoisted our ensign, on purpose to know of her from whence she came, how far she might be from the coast of America, whether she had any fresh provisions to spare or could supply us with any rum and sugar. When we came nigh her we found she was an Irish ship come from Barbadoes bound for Cork in Ireland. We told her our condition, and the master desired us to hoist out our boat, which was immediately done, so our mate and 4 of the sailors went on board of her and were very kindly entertained; but they could not spare us any fresh provisions, only they supplied us with what rum and sugar we wanted. We understood from them she came from Barbadoes on June 4, and reckoned they were about 4 hundred leagues from the coast of America. They likewise told us they left the trade wind in the lat. of 30-00.

July 4. We immediately steer S on purpose to make the trade wind. It is now very hot weather but the sailors can stand it out a little better because we gave them a dram now and then. But our master is very lazy, lying in his bed and getting himself drunk for 2 or 3 days successively, without offering to take one observation or mind the ship's course. We make but slow way, our ship being very foul.

July 5. About 3 in the morning our watch cries for all hands upon deck, at the same time telling there was one of the ship's company fallen overboard. Immediately there was ropes thrown overboard, but all to no purpose, for 'ere the ship could be turned about, he perished. This poor fellow was one of the transports and had a hand in stealing our wine. The day the hottest we have had yet.

July 6. Fair clear weather. We continue to steer to the S. We perceive now a vast many dolphins and flying fish, which we frequently catch and make very good food of them, they being the only fresh provisions we can have.

July 7. Stormy weather. We sail all day long under a reef mainsail; but about 10 at night our master being in liquor, to show his courage, ordered the sailors to hoist the main topsail, then the foresail and foretop-sail, at which the mates showed him the danger whereto he exposed the ship, cargo, and all their lives; but he, being headstrong, ordered them to hoist topgallant sail, which they, by the supercargo's persuasion, refused; and by force hauled him down to his cabin, where they shut him in all night. They lowered the sails presently, yet notwithstanding, the water had got over the gunnel and damaged several parcels of goods.

July 8. Fair clear weather. This day our supercargo takes a protest against the master. About noon we catch a shark 9 foot long, they having continued about our ship ever since our man fell overboard.

From July 9 to 26, we still continue to steer S, in which time we catched a vast many dolphins and bonitos, which was a great preservative against the scurvy, we having nothing but one barrel of salt pork aboard; but the greatest want we labored under now was the want of water, which, though stinking as it was, had all along preserved our lives. We were now reduced to almost one English pint per day, until

July 27, when there fell such a quantity of rain water as would have filled all the vessels we had, if we could have got them soon enough upon deck. We are now in the latitude 31-14.

July 28. We are just coming into the trade wind, but by the master's orders, we are obliged to tack about and steer NW and WNW, by which we could perceive his design was to protract the time as long as he could.

August 4. Pleasant weather. About 8 in the morning we spied a ship to the windward of us about 2 leagues. All our water we had being un-wholesome and our rum gone, we hailed her to see if she could spare us any provisions or fresh water. When she came within speaking, we asked them from whence they came and to whom they belonged. They answered they belonged to Boston in New England, came from Newfoundland, and were bound for South Carolina. We then begged them to spare us what provisions they could, offering any price for them. But they answered they could spare nothing but some salt fish and a little rum, they being very scarce of water and provisions themselves. Then we gave them what they demanded and so parted. We understood by them that they reckoned themselves but 70 leagues from the Capes of Virginia; but to our experi-ence we found afterwards we were more than 4 times 70 distant.

From August 5 to 23, very high winds and for the most part contrary. Here we find very strong currents setting sometimes northerly and then southerly, so that it was very difficult to keep a due reckoning.

August 26. About 10 in the morning perceived a ship about 3 leagues ahead. We hoisted our ensign, at which she bore down to us, and came up with us about 12. She had come from Nevis in the West Indies, had been load with rum, sugar and molasses, but having lost her masts in a hurri-cane, they were obliged to throw most of their rum and sugar overboard. She was steering for New England to repair and have new masts. We could get no help from them, it being then a very high sea.

From August 26 to September 2, very fair winds. We are now quite run out of bread, so that we were obliged to eat peas, but to our great comfort we had still water aboard.

September 3. Spied a ship on our starboard quarter, but it being then a NW[ester], which is a violent NW wind which continues about an hour, we could not speak her until it was over. She was a ship come from New York bound for Surinam in the West Indies, her cargo being most partly [sic] horses, having 29 of them when she came away and now only 12 remaining, being obliged to throw 17 of them overboard by the violence of the weather. We got from them 2 barrels of flour, which was a considerable helping our great necessity. We continued until this time in a pretty good state of health, saving the scurvy, which now began to show its effects upon our men's constitutions, for there was scarce 5 able to work the ship. In this condition we continued until

September 19, which was a day like to have cost us all our lives. It was a violent hurricane which began thus: Early in the morning we perceived a little black cloud rising from the NE. About one hour afterward it rose higher and spread broader. Our mate, who knew what it portended, immediately ordered the sails to be furled and the yards lowered; by the time this was done, we could perceive the cloud coming with mighty force and the sea at a distance rising like the Alps in a mass. It grew terrible dark as it approached, with all the other signs of terror. It was immediately ordered all hands upon deck and with much difficulty 7 came, the rest not being able or willing. We then shut all the hatches very close and secured the boat. The sea now began to be very high, and there was nothing but terror before us: large huge waves breaking over our stern and mizzen mast; our men crying to one another, but not a word to be heard, except they came close to one another's ears and whispered. At last there came a wave, like a mountain, which washed over our main top [shrouds] and brought the ship on her board side. At the same time ballast, goods and all shifted in the hold. Our ship lying on her broad side, made water very fast, and there was no pumping of her, none being able to stand upon deck. At last, with much difficulty, we got 2 men lashed fast to the pump to relieve one another. We had not much hope of our lives but, relying on Providence, the carpenter was ordered to cut away the mizzen mast, which, done, we thought to have likewise cut the main mast, but before they set about it, the violence of the wind blew it off and the main yard, which fell directly upon the gunnel and almost shattered it to pieces. It was indeed very terrible now to see our ship, without either mast or sails, exposed to the violence of a raging sea, and so few hands able to work, so that had it not been the Providence of almighty God, we had all certainly perished. While the carpenter stood ready with his axe, there came a terrible wave, which washed him and 2 others overboard, but they were all 3 taken up alive. This tempest continued from 8 in the morning until 4 in the afternoon, but the height of it did not continue above 3 hours. About 5 we went down to the hold, where we found it much better than expectation, there being not above 2 foot of water in it, but the goods were much damaged. The ship lay all this time on her broad side, so that there was no standing; however, we shifted as well as we could the goods and ballast, and brought the ship a little to rights. Next morning proved a fine day, but it was very dismal to see our ship destitute of masts and sails, we not knowing how far we might be from any land. In the place of a main mast, we set up one old foretop mast, and for the mizzen one oar. We got old rotten remnants of sails in the hold and patched them up as well as we could, and after this manner we continued until the end of our voyage.

About 4 days after this we met a sloop in as bad a condition as ourselves, if not worse. She had met with a violent storm in the month of August, by which she lost her mast and her upper deck and cabin, with the super-cargo in it. They had neither compass nor quadrant aboard and, having lost their rudder, were obliged to let her drive as the winds permitted. They had come from New England and bound for Jamaica. We spared them a compass and quadrant, for which our Captain got 8 barrels of flour and 6 firkins of butter. The weather continued very good and on Sunday,

September 29, we got soundings in 34 fathom water. About 5 after-noon we got sight of North Carolina, which was very acceptable to us, we not having seen land this 6 months and more. This day one of our men fell overboard and one died. Here we anchored 2 days, in which time we run a great hazard of our lives, for there happened at this time to be a Bristol ship and a Maryland ship riding along with us: the Maryland ship had come from Jamaica load with rum, sugar and molasses. The Bristol man came from Guinea but had disposed of his slaves in Barbadoes, and was bound homeward with a cargo of sugar. He had lost all of his men but 5 hands, and this Maryland ship was to conduct him to Virginia, where he was to get more hands and provisions. Our Captain went aboard to see him and there got himself very drunk. It being late at night when he came aboard and high sea, we could not get our boat hoisted in, which occasioned its being lost, for all night the sea was rough and next morning about 10 she was staved to pieces. The weather continued very tempestuous all that day, which forced the Maryland ship to slip her anchor, but the Bristol man and we still kept fast until about 12 at night, when the Bristol ship slipped likewise. Now, if she had struck on our vessel, it had been perhaps the loss of both ships, to save which we were just going to cut our cable, and had already cut it half through when the ship drove by us about 6 yards, and the wind being right on shore, forced the ship against a hard beach, where she was staved to pieces and all in her perished, they being fast asleep when she sliped her anchor. We had gone the same way had it not been for the toughness of our ropes.

Next day the wind proved fair and we weighed anchor and sailed along the coast toward Virginia; but we happened in the night time to sail by the Capes and the wind afterward turning N, we could not get back again. Here we met with an English ship bound for Maryland, from whom we got some fresh provisions, but our gums were so swelled with the scurvy we could scarce eat them. We continued about 2 days, and the third the wind turning fair, we got into the Capes, where, to complete our misfortunes, our Captain through his rashness run the ship aground in the bay, where she still continues without any hope of getting her off. Our whole crew were 19 when we came from Scotland and there are but 14 alive. Thus ends this tedious voyage, which continued 6 months and 17 days, we having come from Scotland April 4, 1728, and entered the Capes of Virginia October 21, 1728.

Cunningham made his way to Williamsburg. The capital town, however, was no place for an impecunious Scot, he thought, even though he could draw on his father for funds and had introductions to such fellow-Scots in that part of Virginia as Alexander Mackenzie of Hampton and Dr. James Blair of the College of William and Mary. In and near this village of " at most " sixty families, Adam wrote his father in 1729, there were " no less than 25 or 30 phisitians, and of that number not above 2 capable of living handsomly." More than this, he went on, the Williamsburg inns, where a bachelor must live, charged exorbitant prices, so that he could not afford to tarry. Accordingly, after providing himself with a stock of medicines, Cunningham travelled " up the country a considerable way," surveying prospects for practice in each county, but everywhere he " either found the parts provided with phisitians or so poor as not [to be] able to maintain one." It was the same story in Maryland. Despairing of establishing himself in America, on Dr. Blair's advice he decided to return to Scotland. Within a few days of the time he was to sail (as ship's surgeon on a vessel leaving the Rappahannock), Cunningham was stricken by an ague. On his recovery he journeyed up the river once more and settled near the Bristol Iron Works in King George's County. It was the sickly season, and he expected business would be brisk.[4]

At the Bristol Iron Works Cunningham was at least busy, even if he did not prosper.

As to my affairs in relation to physick, I cannot much complain, [he told his father in 1730], for I could have works enough of charity, to perform that way almost every day in the year, and indeed I cannot see a poor planter asking my advice or begging my medicines, without being touched with pity, and freely give him away the drugs that have cost me above

---

[4] Adam Cunningham to Sir William Cunningham, King George's County, Va., August 2, 1729.

150 per cent in this country. I must own I do my endeavor to make it up with the richer sort, but these gentlemen are so very careful not to fall sick, as I almost despair of making any thing of them. This is indeed, Sir, the truth of the matter, and in my humble opinion there is no way of making money in this country so easy as by merchandizing, this being the occupation they all come at, for after they have purchased a little stock by their practice, they presently commence merchants, and so make their fortune. So that if Doctor Blair, Colonel McKenzie, and many others whom I could name have made their fortunes in this country, it is not to be attributed to their practice in physick but to traffick.[5]

Neither by physick nor traffick did Cunningham make his fortune. When he quit Virginia and returned home is not known. But from Newcastle-upon-Tyne, travelling from London to Edinburgh in the late winter of 1735-1736, he wrote his father to beg for money and arrange a secret rendezvous. He was in serious trouble and could not see friends or family. At least Adam spoke of his going abroad again as being for his father's honor and his own safety, and he expressed the hope that he might " be transported from Port Glasgow to some of the foreign plantations where I may pass the remainder of my days in a sincere repentence of my former folly." [6]

Nothing more than this is known of Adam Cunningham. The family tradition is that he disappeared in Virginia, perhaps after a second passage of the ocean as stormy as the one whose record his family still preserve.

[5] Same to same, Bristol Mines, Va., May 24, 1730.
[6] Same to same, Newcastle-upon-Tyne, March 23, 1736.

William Shippen, Jr.'s Introductory Lecture, 1762

The Medical School of the College of Philadelphia was enveloped in personal controversy and rivalry from the moment of its founding in 1765. John Morgan, the first professor to be appointed, in his inaugural *Discourse upon the Institution of Medical Schools in America,* referred condescendingly to Dr. William Shippen, Jr., who had been teaching anatomy as a private instructor for the past three years, and intimated that he would be an acceptable addition to the faculty. Shippen, who was in fact named professor of anatomy soon afterwards, took the occasion of his course announcement in 1766 to refer to, and quote from, his introductory lecture in the State House in 1762 for the purpose of establishing his priority. No record of what Shippen actually said appears to have survived.

A second account, somewhat fuller than Shippen's, has now come to light. Written by one of the audience, probably a young man, certainly a Quaker, it seems to have been prepared as an exercise in attention and composition. Someone interested in the Medical School, perhaps a partisan of one of the antagonists, appears to have seen the report and asked for a copy—which is what the manuscript here published appears to be. Neither the author nor the recipient is named.

Although the document has some interest because of the importance of the episode to which it relates, it lacks the greatest significance because it says nothing conclusive on the point that was at issue between Morgan and Shippen— whether the latter did in fact intend to establish a medical school on a collegiate base.

The document is in the Charles Roberts Autograph Collection (Box 231) in the Haverford College Library, Haverford, Pennsylvania. The full text follows:

Respected Friend

I now send thee a Sketch of what was proposed to me as an Exercise.

I did not care to be too particular lest other Business should obstruct my Intention.

The inditing &c: has employd me about two Hours since Breakfast, and therefore may be judg'd of in Conformity.

Philadelphia Novr: 17th: 1762

Last Night William Shippen Junr: appear'd at the State House in a publick Lecture on the Advantages accruing from the Knowledge of the human Frame, not only to such whose particular Callings rendered it absolutely necessary to them, but likewise to several other Branches of civil Society.

He introduc'd his Discourse by an Apology for himself, intimating his Consciousness of his Incapacity for his present Undertaking, but in Consideration of it's extensive Usefulnes, & encourag'd by his worthy Patron Doctor Fothergill, by the noted Doctor Hunter under whom he studied, as well as by all his Friends both here & in England, he was determined to lay aside all that Diffidence so natural to a young Man and apply with chearfulness to the Task intended.

He then proceeded with a brief Account of the Progress of Anatomy for many Centurys. He mentioned the Butcher as Author of some Discoveries, as well as enumerated the Names of such particular Students in this Science as have left behind them more remarkable Observations: Among the Rest he renown'd the famous Harvey, whose Illucidations respecting the Circulation of the Blood would transmit his Name to late Posterity.

In the Course of his Lecture, he spoke of the particular Necessity of this Knowledge to Gentlemen who attempted to administer to the Wants of their afflicted Neighbors, and introduc'd some familiar Instances to impress the Force of what was mention'd.

Says he, there's a certain Pain in the Shoulder which as it proceeds from the Liver, how is it possible that any Man who does not understand the Connections between those two Parts can apply a proper Remedy: And further, who having a Watch that is out of Order would trust her for a Regulation to such a One as he is certain is not acquainted with the Intestine Parts.

He then inform'd his Audience with the Method he intended to pursue in the Instruction of his Pupils. He would begin with that great & material Part the Blood, then the Bones &c: afterwards with Dissection & Bandages, and between Whiles would introduce a small Part of Physiology, but upon the Arrival of his Friend & fellow Citizen, John Morgan, he would readily resign that Branch & refer his Pupils to his further Instruction.

Then, To such who would attempt the Art he gave an Instance of great Encouragement. He informd them that 50 Years agoe Edinburgh that renowned Seminary was nothing, that Doctor Monro was the first who read Lectures there and is now living, and excited them to persevere with the following Exhortation—Who knows but the Honor of further Improvements is reserv'd for this young tho' growing & flourishing Country.

Thus to investigate Nature & find the Causes of her several Operations may be of infinite Benefit to Mankind, be particularly serviceable to the Country, and put it in the Power of skilful Persons to save the Lives of Numbers, who otherwise might meet their Fate by trusting in dangerous Cases to the Hands of Ignorance.

Postscript

We descended to many other Particulars to show the wonderful Mechanism constituting the human Frame, and in the Course of his Observations on the Propriety of every Part he justly remarkd upon the Wisdom of the mighty Author, & was of Opinion that an Examination into Nature was a Species of Theology and would give more noble Ideas of the great Creator.

Let any Man (says he) undertake in his Imagination to make a Man, he will say perhaps, what need is there of all this extraordinary Apparatus? why would not a less delicate, a less expensive Structure answer the End as well? why? since his Stay here is of so short Duration & his Frame to subject to decay, why shall the Machine be so contrivd, so wonderfully and surprisingly made? But then let him scrutinize the Parts, let him observe the Dependance & Connections thoroughly subsisting, let him behold the surprising Order from Head to Foot and see whether he could change any Particular for the better: Then let him ask himself, is there no Use for this? is there no Service for the other? and will he not conclude, that 'Man's as perfect as he ought,' that by infinite Wisdom he has been created, and that nothing short can add or lessen with advantage to the Beauty or Convenience of the stately Fabric.

Body-Snatching in Philadelphia

The first professor of anatomy in almost every medical school in 18th-
and early 19th-century America had to face charges, usually verbal but
sometimes delivered by armed mobs, that he engaged in grave-robbing to
get materials for classroom dissections. William Shippen, Jr. (1736-1808) in
Philadelphia had this experience. George W. Norris in his *Early History of
Medicine in Philadelphia* relates that Shippen's anatomical class was once
disrupted by a mob and that several times the professor had to conceal himself for safety. In 1770 the familiar charges were renewed; and elicited an
explanation and defense. Though Shippen unequivocally denied taking
bodies from "the Burying-ground of any Denomination of Christians," he
might have taken them—as he once admitted—from the Potter's Field. The
notice reprinted below appeared in the *Pennsylvania Gazette* of 11 January
1770.

WHITFIELD J. BELL, JR.

To the PUBLIC

Many of the Inhabitants of this City, I hear, have been much terrified by sundry wicked and malicious Reports of my taking up Bodies
from the several Burying-grounds in this Place; notwithstanding these
Fears are groundless, the Reports false, and seem either made and
propagated by weak and prejudiced Persons, or intended to injure my
Character, yet *Humanity* obliges me to suppress all Feelings of Resentment and Contempt, and do all in my Power to remove these, tho'
groundless, Fears; which I do, by declaring, in the most solemn Manner, that I never have had, and that I never will have, directly or indirectly, one Subject from the Burying-ground belonging to any Denomination of Christians whatever.—Having been informed that two
Families were very lately much terrified, by unkind Insinuations, that
their deceased Friends would not rest in their Graves, I waited on
them, with a sincere Desire to relieve their distressed Minds, and made
no Doubt but I should receive such Information from them, as would
enable me to trace these black Stories to their blacker Original; but
after the most diligent Enquiry, not one Author could be found, and
all, yes! all these terrible Fears, all this Belief of these wicked and
foolish, nay, almost impossible Stories, depended, as a Gentleman
sensibly expressed it himself, on mere *Fama clamosa, impertinent
noisy Fame;* and all the Information I could get was, that it was generally believed I had taken up a young Lady from Christ-Church
Burying-ground, whose Grave has been opened within these few Days,
and her Body found in its sacred Repository undisturbed. And sec-
ondly, that scarce any one doubted but I had in my Theatre the Body
of Elizabeth Roberts, who formerly lived as House-keeper with William Lyons, Esq; this Woman, as Dr. Kearsley jun. (who attended her
in her last Illness) has given me from under his Hand, died in the
Middle of Summer of a putrid Fever, yet no one doubts but I dissected
her in the Middle of Winter. By such inconsistent, such false Stories,

have some of your Minds, my Fellow Citizens, been much alarmed, and my Character and Usefulness, essentially injured. May I not flatter myself, your Resentment against me will be turned into Pity, and you will join with me, in endeavouring to discover, and bring to condign Punishment, the wicked Disturbers of your Peace, and Defamers of my Reputation? I have persevered in teaching this difficult and most useful Branch of medical Knowledge, tho' attended with very disagreeable Circumstances, chiefly from the Motive of public Good, and have, and always will preserve the utmost Decency, with regard to the Dead; and do again solemnly protest, that none of your House, or Kindred, shall ever be disturbed in their silent Graves, by me, or any under my Care. As it has been insinuated, that Subjects might have been brought from these Burial Places by my Pupils, without my Knowledge, I have added an Affidavit of Joseph Harrison, Student of Medicine, who has lived in my Father's House ever since I began my anatomical Lectures, and who has had an Opportunity of knowing where every Body was obtained, that ever I dissected in America.

W. SHIPPEN, jun. *Professor of Anatomy*

City of Philadelphia, ss.

On the Fifth Day of January, in the Year of our Lord One Thousand Seven Hundred and Seventy, before us, Samuel Shoemaker, Esq; Mayor, and Isaac Jones, Esq; one of the Aldermen of this City, personally appeared Joseph Harrison, of the said City, Student of Physic, and being sworn on the Holy Evangelists of Almighty GOD, did depose and say, That he has lived with Dr. Shippen, sen. as an Apprentice, for eight Years last past, and has regularly attended every Course of anatomical Lectures, exhibited by Dr. Shippen, jun. and has had an Opportunity of seeing, and, to the best of this Deponent's Knowledge and Belief, has seen every Subject that has been dissected by the said Dr. Shippen, jun. and knows with Certainty, how, and from what Place, every such Subject was obtained; and upon his said Oath does say and declare, that not one of said Subjects, which this Deponent has seen dissected, or procured to be dissected, was taken out of any Burying-ground belonging to any religious Society in this City; and doth further say and depose, that there never was, to this Deponent's Knowledge, any dead Body taken from any of the aforesaid Burying-grounds to be dissected by any other Person whatsoever, and has good Reason to believe, no such Thing could have been done by any of the Students of Anatomy, without his Knowledge, since Dr. Shippen began his Lectures.

JOSEPH HARRISON.

Sworn the Day and Year above mentioned, before
SAMUEL SHOEMAKER, Mayor.
ISAAC JONES.

An Eighteenth Century
American Medical Manuscript
The Clinical Notebook of John Archer, M.B., 1768

THE medical notes in manuscript of John Archer, 1768M, recently presented to the University of Pennsylvania Library, are documents which add details and some new facts to our knowledge of the history of medicine in the United States. Kept by a member of the first class of the first medical school in North America, the notes tell a good deal directly and indirectly about the conditions and quality of medical practice and the content of medical education at a time when some American physicians were trying to raise professional standards and establish medical schools in America. Incidentally but specifically, the notes are important to biographers of Dr. John Morgan, 1757C, of Dr. Thomas Bond, and, of course, of John Archer.[1]

Born in what is now Harford County, Maryland, in 1741, John Archer was sent to West Nottingham Academy, where John Morgan and William Shippen, Jr., had preceded him and Benjamin Rush was a fellow student. He was graduated at the College of New Jersey at Princeton in 1760, in the same class with Rush. Young Archer announced an intention of opening an academy in Baltimore. He seems not to have done so, however, and shortly afterward began to study for the ministry. He revealed "such a want of knowledge in divinity & the other particulars he has been examined on, as well as such an incapacity to communicate his ideas on any subject," that the Presbytery rejected him for ordination. In the summer of 1765 Archer came to Philadelphia to study medicine as John Morgan's apprentice.[2]

Dr. Morgan had just begun his professional career with an éclat unparalleled in America. Reports of his astonishing academic and social successes in Europe had preceded him to Philadelphia: he had been made a Fellow of the Royal Society and of the Royal College of Physicians of Edinburgh and had traveled in Italy with the Duke of York and visited Voltaire at Ferney. Within a few days of his return he was elected Professor of Medicine in the College of Philadelphia. A month later, on May 30, 1765, in a *Discourse on the Institution of Medical Schools in America*, Morgan laid down what he considered a sound program of practice and education. To popular fame Morgan quickly added professional reputation; by late summer he had a practice, and physicians and laymen alike were consulting him by mail in difficult cases.

"I am daily at Dr. Morgan's shop," Archer wrote his fiancée in the winter of 1765–66, "& on Mondays, Wednesdays, & Fridays attend his Lectures [on theory and practice]—the Course is four Pistoles & a Dollar [for the library]. Tuesdays, Thursdays & Saturdays Dr. Shippen's [on anatomy]—the course Six Pistoles." In addition, as Archer's student notes show, he attended Dr. Thomas Bond's clinical lectures at the Pennsylvania Hospital. "I have concluded to remain in Philadelphia," he wrote, "until Spring come a year."

As Morgan's apprentice Archer compounded medicines, accompanied his master on visits to the sick and sometimes attended them alone, and was allowed and encouraged to copy exchanges of letters from Morgan's consulting practice. These exchanges, as well as more formal essays, constitute the bulk of the material in the volume which the Library has now acquired. Written at different times over a two-year period, the folios were bound up to form a kind of clinical casebook. The volume contains upwards of 200 pages. Writing appears on the right-hand leaves, except for a few corrections and additions on left-hand pages.

The case records are all from Morgan's practice in 1766–67. Morgan is certainly the author of "A True Peripneumony," and is probably the author of other essays as well. The questions and answers on physiology are based on Morgan's course, and may have been asked in a public examination. On the other hand, the report of a post-mortem in which a polypus was found in the right ventricle of the heart, is Bond's. Archer himself was the author of an address to a student medical society, which is the last item in the volume.[3]

Not only are the case records interesting in themselves; they throw light on medical practice. John Potts' wife had been troubled for months by irregular menstruation; her husband (who was the father of one of Morgan's pupils) asked Morgan's professional advice. In Fredericksburg, Virginia, Hugh Mercer, whom Morgan knew ten years before when both served in the army on the Pennsylvania frontier, had a patient with a persistent skin tumor. Morgan found the case so puzzling that he submitted it to the Philadelphia Medical Society (which he had founded), and forwarded Mercer their diagnosis and prescriptions—warm baths, ointment, medicines and a regular diet.[4]

Both Morgan's prescriptions in particular cases and his more general essays reveal him as a cautious practitioner, putting his trust in diet, fresh air, and the healing power of the Yellow Springs in Chester County, quite as much as in medicines. "Diet is a Cooperator with Medicine in the Cure of Disease," he declared. "Yet let us not despair," he wrote in a discussion of pulmonary tuberculosis,

softly & easy goes far; festina lente is a Motto truly applicable here. No Time is to be lost in the Use of the most bland, safe & efficacious Medicines & they must be resolutely persisted in. A strong Enemy deeply entrenched is in Possession of the Citadel: a violent assault will sooner demolish the City, than compel such an Enemy to surrender. Here we want the City entire, which is easier gained by a steady, resolute & artful Conduct, than by placing all Hopes on a Rash tho' powerful Attack.

In the same spirit Morgan observed to his students

that Nature is the Physician & we only her Assistants, waiting with diligence to embrace her Indications, to strengthen her when weak, to correct her when too violent & even to shew her the most salutary Way when hesitating, that Death may be disappointed pro tempore & the Sick restored to health & Vigor again.

Quite as important as what Archer's notes tell of medical practice in eighteenth-century America is what they tell of medical education during the first years the medical department of the College of Philadelphia was in existence. The opportunities for post-mortems, for example, were few; when one presented itself the students seized it.

A certain James Richardson last 7*ber* [September] was suddenly seized with an Asthma, or Difficulty of Breathing, which daily encreased; he was also some Time after taken with a Pleurisy, of which he recovered; but still retained his former Complaint—he became Anasarcous in his lower Extremities to a considerable Degree: the upper not being much affected. . . . On the 23d of April [1766] he made Application, & was admitted into the Pennsylvania Hospital under the Care of Dr. Thomas Bond, the then attending Physician, who examined him particular, as to those Symptoms already noted, & what we shall further observe. Upon a further enquiry of his Case he related, that he could not ly on any Side, but the Left & his Back, and in setting up he found the greatest Ease, which was his Posture Day and Night. Further this other Circumstance may be worthy our Notice in accounting for the Phaenomena: he was given to excess in the Use of Spirituous Liquors—*Women* & *Wine* the two Outlets to Man's Ruin. Again he was observed to evacuate clotted Blood at his Mouth & Nose every Night. . . .

Prognosis—After enquiring into the above particulars Dr. Bond did not hesitate to declare, that he was certain, there was an Obstruction occasioned by a Polypus either in the Heart or Pulmonary Artery.

On Saturday the 26th inst. he died suddenly. From the above Prognosis a Desire of Improvement excited the attending Students to have the Body opened, which was accordingly done. . . .

Then follow the post-mortem findings in detail, with the final statement:

For a more particular Satisfaction of Curiosity & your Improvement I refer you to the Polypus which is deposited in the Pennsylvania Hospital among many other Curiosities equally curious.

Post-mortems such as this enriched the formal curriculum of lectures and demonstrations. So did the exchange of information and opinion in what Archer's notes call "the Hospital Medical Society." This was presumably the first student medical society in North America. Patterned on the student societies at Edinburgh, where Dr. Morgan was a member of the Medical (later Royal Medical) Society, "the Hospital Medical Society" at Philadelphia was composed of students regularly enrolled in Bond's course and, possibly, of apprentices not studying for a degree at the College. Archer may have been the Society's first president. In any event, in January or February 1767 he addressed the members on their purposes and opportunities.[5]

Each Member is by the Rules of this Society to write a Medical Thoesies [sic] in his Turn on any Subject, he thinks himself most capable to discuss. From this will arise many Advantages, as not only the Tho'ts he has already of the Nature of the Disorder, its Indications and Cure will be regularly arranged; but he will be immediately entred on a careful Scrutiny of the most approved Authors, who have wrote on the Subject, & will consequently adopt the most rational & practical Observations, & imprint them on his Mind. . . . Altho' this advantage may appear to be particularly adapted to one Person; yet when we consider, that all are obliged to write in their Turn, it becomes common—

Again, this Theosis is to be read publickly at our appointed Meeting, which will be a great Advantage to every individual of this Society, as each Thoesis will be a theoretico-practical Treatise on the particular Subject he has chosen, whether of Physic or Chirurgery. By this Method we shall be able to discriminate Disorders, their Natures, Indications & Cures. From this we will not only have an Oppertunity to lay up many useful Remarks in our common medical Treasury; but also have many others revived, that were almost sunk in Oblivion.

Another Advantage not less than those already mentioned is our Improvement in Writing on Medical Subjects—There are many Physicians who may be said to understand Disorders & their Treatment; yet are unable to communicate their Sentiments with Perspicuity in writing when required, or necessity obliges them to communicate the Case to any of the Faculty.

Again, should any of us from being Juniors explicate Disorders improperly, or indistinctly point out their Inductions, & an injudicial Method of Treatment from such a collective Body we promise ourselves Mistakes (if any) would not pass Unnoticed; but be observed with friendly Eyes & therefore be rationally rectified.

A few months after he read this address to his fellow-students Archer left Philadelphia to begin practice. He had hoped to practice with an older man in Lancaster, Pennsylvania, but this intention was frustrated. "Therefore," he wrote his wife on April 21, 1767, "I still have the wide world to seek where to pitch my tent." He pitched it in Delaware, first at Hamburg, then at St. George's. His books show that he charged the usual fees (bleeding, 2/6, inoculation, £1, tooth extraction, 2/6, visits 5/– and 1/– a mile for every mile over five, with night calls at 10/–) and that he was sometimes paid, after the custom of rural Delaware, in pork, potatoes, cordwood, even a pair of shoes for his Negro servant.

In the spring of 1767 the Trustees of the College of Philadelphia adopted a plan to award degrees of Bachelor and Doctor of

Medicine. Archer was examined the next year, and qualified for his M.B. Nine other young physicians did likewise. On June 21, 1768, the ten men were graduated Bachelors of Medicine. By accident of alphabet John Archer's name stood first in the list of those who were graduated on what Provost William Smith proudly hailed as "the birthday of Medical honors in America."

Probably it was at this time that Archer was offered, but declined, a partnership with John Morgan in Philadelphia. He stayed in Delaware until 1769 when he returned to Harford County, where he practised more than 40 years until his death. Occasionally during that time he wrote a scientific paper, often on some wonder. Someone brought him a kind of amphibious creature; he stuffed it and sent it with a description to the American Philosophical Society. The men who chased and killed the beast, Archer explained, declared "that it was very active & springy as it did when persued leap five or six Yards on level Ground. Those who killed it thot that it made the most use of its Tail in Leaping."[6] In several medical papers he reported medical marvels, like the case of a woman who, having intercourse with a white man and a Negro successively, gave birth to twins, one white, the other black.[7]

Archer's other papers, based on his practical experience, were less astonishing. Whooping-cough, he reported, could be checked by vaccination. He had success in treating patients with intermittent fevers by dosing them before, rather than after, the attacks. He is said to have devised a method of reducing fractures which Philip Syng Physick independently developed later.[8]

For these things John Archer would be remembered. But his greatest distinction as a physician is that, at the home he built in Harford County and called Medical Hall, he trained about 50 young men in his profession. Four of his six sons became doctors and a fifth was studying medicine under his father when the boy died. At Medical Hall in 1797 Archer formed the Harford County Medical Society. Six of its eight members were Archers. As in the "Hospital Medical Society" 30 years before, each member read in his turn "a dissertation corroborating or confuting some medical opinion which influences the Practice of Physic," or a paper on one of the sciences related to medicine.[9]

John Archer died in 1810. His sons and grandsons who lived in Harford County were physicians, judges, and members of Congress. They inherited Archer's medical memorabilia, and ultimately gave many to the Medical and Chirurgical Faculty of Maryland (of which John Archer was a founder in 1799). One son went to Mississippi and he inherited the volume of clinical notes his father had made in Philadelphia in 1766–1767. After almost 200 years those notes have now been returned as a gift of the Class of 1916M to the Medical School of whose graduates John Archer was the first and surely not the least useful.

NOTES

1. The manuscript was presented to the University by the Class of 1916M in honor of their member John G. Archer, of Greenville, Miss., the great-great-grandson of the writer of the medical notes.

2. The principal biographical sketches of John Archer are by "one of his descendants" in the *Bulletin of the Johns Hopkins Hospital*, X (1899): 141–47, and by J. Alexis Shriver in the *Bulletin of the Medical Library Association*, XX (1932): 90–101. Archer's medical ledger, 1775–1783, his notes on Materia Medica taken in Dr. Adam Kuhn's course, 1767–1768, his arts and medical diplomas, and other memorabilia are preserved in the library of the Medical and Chirurgical Faculty of Maryland, Baltimore.

3. The volume contains the following material: An essay on crisis, based on Hippocrates.—Obstruction.—An essay on inflammatory fevers.—A true peripneumony.—A dissertation on a phthisis pulmonalis.—De urinis.—A relation of a polypus in the right ventricle of the heart.—A case of cutaneous eruptive tumors of an infectious nature.—A case.—De usu et abusu concubitus.—A case of an irregular flow of the menses.—A case of obstructed menses.—Directions to be observed in treating the cholic.—A case of uterine haemorrhage. —Questions and answers on physiology.—Address to "the Hospital Medical Society."

    Some of these case records were also copied in the notes of one of Archer's classmates, Jonathan Elmer, who names Morgan as the author of "A True Peripneumony," (cf. Elmer, *Miscellania Medica*, manuscript in the possession of the late Dr. Robert P. Elmer, Wayne, Pa.)

4. Hugh Mercer to John Morgan, May 16, 1767, Dreer Collection, *Generals of the American Revolution*, II: 41, Historical Society of Pennsylvania; same to same, June 22, 1767, University of Virginia.

5. The manuscript is torn. One can read only "Pennsylvania Hospital
   (. . .)ary 27, 1767.

6. John Archer to Dr. Robert Harris, December 2, 1773. *Ms. Communications*, I:6, American Philosophical Society.

7. "An Inflammation, apparently of the Ovarium, ending in Suppura-
   tion, and discharging a living worm and a well shaped tooth. (With
   the tooth);" and "Facts illustrating a Disease peculiar to the female
   children of Negro Slaves: and Observations, showing that a white
   woman by intercourse with a white man and a Negro, may conceive
   twins, one of which shall be white, and the other a mulatto . . . ,"
   Medical Repository, XII (1809):365–66; XIII (1810):319–23.

8. "The Hooping-Cough cured by Vaccination," *ibid.*, XII (1809):
   182–83; "A Biographical Sketch of John Archer, M.B.," *Medical and
   Surgical Reporter*, XXII (1870):129–31. See also Archer's "Case of
   extraordinary recovery from wounded stomach . . . ," communicated by his son to the *Medical Repository*, XV (1812):215–17.

9. The manuscript transactions of the Society are in the library of the
   Medical and Chirurgical Faculty of Maryland, Baltimore. They are
   commented on by Eugene F. Cordell in the *Bulletin of the Johns
   Hopkins Hospital*, XIII (1902):181–88.

   During the American Revolution Archer was politically active in
   the American cause, and in 1801–1807 he was a member of Congress. Walter W. Preston, *History of Harford County, Maryland*, Baltimore, 1901, pp. 96, 101–102, 106–107, 201; Peter Force, ed.,
   American Archives, 4th ser.,IV:737; 5th ser.,II:637.

Dr. James Rush on his Philadelphia, Edinburgh, and London Teachers

Dr. James Rush (1786-1869), son of the great Benjamin, is generally known, when he is remembered at all, as an early and original student of psychology, the husband of one of Philadelphia's great hostesses, and the author of a will remarkable even in Philadelphia for eccentricity. He was undoubtedly able, intelligent, and accomplished in many respects; but he was also peevish and prickly, with little love or understanding for his fellows. He accepted membership in the American Philosophical Society in 1827, for example, but resigned ten days later when he learned that the Society had also elected Dr. John Kearsley Mitchell, who, Rush charged, had pursued "a course of conduct . . . towards me, alike unprovoked and ungenerous" and was guilty of an "outrageous violation of medical decorum, by a rude intrusion on my professional concerns." Rush thought himself unappreciated by his contemporaries, as he undoubtedly was; and his life more and more dropped away into that of a lonely, embittered recluse.

Young Rush had the same professional training his father had had. After being graduated from Princeton, he went to the University of Pennsylvania, where he received his M.D. in 1809, and then to Edinburgh and London. On returning to Philadelphia in 1811, he practised for a time and read his father's lectures to private classes for four years after Benjamin's death in 1813. He was never elected to the medical faculty of the University, however, or to that of any other Philadelphia medical school.

Rush kept his tickets of admission to medical classes at Pennsylvania, Edinburgh, and London, and years afterwards wrote on the back of each a short characterization of the lecturer. Whether these estimates are in every case accurate and fair is debatable, but there can be little doubt that they clearly reflect a facet of the author's personality.

The tickets are preserved in James Rush's papers in the Library Company of Philadelphia, where they were found by the director, Edwin Wolf 2nd, who has recently given us a short sketch of Rush's character in the Library Company's *Annual Report . . . 1961* (Philadelphia, 1962), pp. 9-19. They are presented here with Mr. Wolf's permission.

UNIVERSITY OF PENNSYLVANIA, 1808-9.

Benjamin Smith Barton [Materia Medica; Botany]. A mass of affectation & vanity, a large burden of ill temper, a little heap of knowledge, and not a mite of genius though altogether matter enough in mind to have bred it.

Philip Syng Physick [Surgery, with Dorsey]. An instance of how a man may grip on to the opinions of the world, without having any claims for it.

John Syng Dorsey [Surgery, with Physick]. A vain man, with common ability and education, got into a place that even he could not have expected. We know what this makes of such a man.

Alexander Ramsay [Anatomy and Physiology]. This Alexander Ramsay was a little, big headed—crooked spined—ham bo shined [bow shinned?] short legged—abortive, rickett spoiled quack of a philosopher who, as a painter's boy was employed to paint the anatomical theatre at Edinburgh, and thinking himself cut out for an anatomist, took up the study; came to Philadelphia in 1807 and delivered a course of foolishness. He was a good specimen of bodily, mental and moral distortion.

Benjamin Rush [Institutes and Practice of Medicine]. Posterity shall know this man.

James Woodhouse [Chemistry]. Some men will get to be professors, and you cannot tell why.

UNIVERSITY OF EDINBURGH, 1809-10.

Charles Hope [Chemistry and Pharmacy]. A very neat and successful experimenter—and a *nice* gentleman.

Alexander Monro Sr. [i.e., *secundus*. Anatomy and Surgery, with Monro Jr.]. He show'd me volumes of his Cases record in detail—and not a leaf of deduction. Very laborious!

Alexander Monro Jr. [i.e., *tertius*. Anatomy and Surgery, with Monro Sr.]. Compared with his place, an Idiot.

John Murray [Materia Medica and Pharmacy]. Too fluent in speech to admit this conclusion, that he possessed much comprehensiveness of thought, or breadth of association.

John Thomson [Military Surgery; Surgery]. A very worthy man— better perhaps than many with more fame. He seemed to work hard among learning to try to do some thing. But he never seem'd able to raise his own head above the chaos of books about him.

Dugald Stewart [Moral Philosophy]. A most respectable and learned man—with more character than ability.

LONDON

Charles Bell [Anatomy and Surgery]. Of this gentleman I thought more highly than of any of the Medical profession whose lectures I attended in Britain. He lectur'd unconnected with any Institution, and his class was about *eighteen!!*—whilst many asses in place at the several Hospitals had benches to overflowing. It pleas'd me to leave the mob and go to him.

Astley Cooper [Surgery]. A very great surgeon, as they always say of some one in a city, with much affectation. A Dandy in speech and thought and manner.

Everard Home [St. George's Hospital]. Had such an itch for discovery that he did nothing but tickle his own vanity with conceits of originality.

On a ticket of admission to lectures on "Institutes and Practice of Medicine, by the late Dr. Benjamin Rush, read by his son Dr. James Rush," the latter wrote: "I read the Lectures of Dr. B. Rush for four courses—viz. 1813, 1814, 1815, 1816, when I gave it up—The class dwindling to almost my merely private pupils—The opposition of the University of Pennsylvania and the aristocratic tyranny around it being too strong for me and my father's lectures into the bargain."

Library of Congress Cataloging in Publication Data

Bell, Whitfield Jenks.
　　The colonial physician & other essays.

　　CONTENTS: Portrait of the colonial physician.
—Philadelphia medical students in Europe, 1750-
1800.—John Redman, medical preceptor (1722-1808).
—Thomas Parke, physician and friend. [etc.]
　　1. Medicine—United States—History. 2. Medicine—Pennsylvania—Philadelphia—History. 3. Medicine—Pennsylvania—Philadelphia—Biography.
4. Medicine—15th-18th centuries. I. Title.
[DNLM: 1. History of medicine, 18th century—Pennsylvania—Essays. 2. Physicians—Pennsylvania—
Biography. WZ140 AP4 B4c]

Library of Congress Cataloging in Publication Data

R152.B43　　610'.9748'11　　75-6652
ISBN 0-88202-024-2